THE BODY
SCOOP
FOR GIRLS

THE BODY SCOOP

FOR GIRLS

A Straight-Talk Guide to a Healthy, Beautiful You

JENNIFER ASHTON, M.D., OB-GYN

with Christine Larson

AVERY

a member of Penguin Group (USA) Inc.

New York

AVERY

Published by the Penguin Group

Penguin Group (USA) Inc., 375 Hudson Street, New York, New York 10014,
USA · Penguin Group (Canada), 90 Eglinton Avenue East, Suite 700,
Toronto, Ontario M4P 2Y3, Canada (a division of Pearson Penguin Canada Inc.) · Penguin
Books Ltd, 80 Strand, London WC2R 0RL, England · Penguin Ireland, 25 St Stephen's
Green, Dublin 2, Ireland (a division of Penguin Books Ltd) · Penguin Group (Australia),
250 Camberwell Road, Camberwell, Victoria 3124, Australia (a division of Pearson Australia
Group Pty Ltd) · Penguin Books India Pvt Ltd, 11 Community Centre, Panchsheel Park,
New Delhi-110 017, India · Penguin Group (NZ), 67 Apollo Drive, Rosedale, North Shore
0632, New Zealand (a division of Pearson New Zealand Ltd) · Penguin Books (South Africa)
(Pty) Ltd, 24 Sturdee Avenue, Rosebank, Johannesburg 2196, South Africa

Penguin Books Ltd, Registered Offices: 80 Strand, London WC2R 0RL, England

Most Avery books are available at special quantity discounts for bulk purchase for
sales promotions, premiums, fund-raising, and educational needs. Special books or
book excerpts also can be created to fit specific needs. For details, write Penguin
Group (USA) Inc. Special Markets, 375 Hudson Street, New York, NY 10014.

Library of Congress Cataloging-in-Publication Data

Ashton, Jennifer.
The body scoop for girls: a straight-talk guide to a healthy, beautiful you /
Jennifer Ashton; with Christine Larson.
            p.   cm.
ISBN 978-1-58333-369-3
1. Teenage girls—Health and hygiene.   2. Puberty.   I. Larson, Christine.   II. Title.
RA777.25.A84   2009   2009036190
        613'.04243—dc22

Printed in the United States of America
1   3   5   7   9   10   8   6   4   2

This book is printed on acid-free paper. ∞

BOOK DESIGN BY NICOLE LAROCHE

CONTENTS

SECTION THREE

·····································

YOUR BODY'S LIFETIME WARRANTY: STAYING HEALTHY FOR LIFE

WHAT TO EXPECT WHEN YOU'RE ADOLESCENT

CHAPTER 1

NOT YOUR MOTHER'S GYNECOLOGIST

You're a New Kind of Girl—You Deserve a New Kind of Medicine

Casey,[1] fifteen, a slender redhead with a sprinkle of freckles on her nose, was sitting next to my desk, twisting a strand of long, straight hair when I walked into my office. I could tell she was nervous.

"Hi, I'm Dr. Ashton," I said, sitting down at my desk. Since this was Casey's first visit, we were meeting in my cheerful office, not in an exam room. (After all, do *you* want to meet your doctor for the very first time in an exam room with your clothes off? I wouldn't either. So my patients meet me in their clothes, at my desk.)

Casey looked startled when I introduced myself. "Really? No way," she burst out. Then she blushed. "Sorry, it's just . . . you don't *look* like a doctor."

I laughed. I hear this all the time. Is it my blond hair? My leopard-print skirt and Tory Burch boots? Lucky for me, I didn't have to check my fashion sense at the door when they were handing out degrees at Columbia Med School. Or my sense of humor, either.

And it's a good thing, too. Without a sincere appreciation for a witty comment or the latest color in Uggs, my job wouldn't be nearly so much fun. I love the humor, the sass, the street sense, and the totally exhilarating energy of my teenage patients. Although I do treat adult women, too (often the mothers of my teen patients), I spend most of my time every day talking with, laughing with, and treating girls from their early teens to early twenties.

That's what Casey and I did—talk and laugh. After a good chuckle over her confusion, we found ourselves talking about pretty much everything—why she'd come (bad cramps), her overall health (pretty good), and her life in general (crazy busy, with dance team practice, SAT prep courses, college visits, and a long-time boyfriend). The more we talked about her incredibly full life, the more Casey reminded me of something—the single most important thing I've learned from my patients. It's this:

It is much, *much* harder to be a teenage girl now than ever before.

Yeah, I know, the lonely-zitty-anxious-harassed teen years have never exactly been an all-expense-paid vacation to Hawaii. But it's tougher today than ever. Even tougher than when I was a teen (and that wasn't *so* long ago—really!). And also tougher, at least in some ways, than when your parents were teens. Sure, you've got your iPod, your cell phone, your computer. You can text your best friend about tomorrow's math test and check your new crush's Facebook page at the same time with one hand tied behind your back. You're smarter, more sophisticated, and way more connected than your parents were (or are). But you're also under phenomenal pressure—academic, social, physical, and sexual.

"You're supposed to get perfect grades, but even straight A's aren't enough to get you into a good college," Casey told me. "You're supposed to volunteer, play sports, and be a genius at something, like violin or math." Don't forget being pretty, popular, and fun. And talk about social pressure—who knows what your so-called friends might be texting about you at any given moment? Sure, social pressure's been around forever. But today it's nonstop, always-on, 24-7.

I asked Casey if she was sexually active. "No," she said. "But at school there's definitely pressure to dress sexy and act like you're having sex."

Where does all this extra sexual pressure come from? *Everywhere.* One study showed that teens today may be exposed to *twice* as much sexual content on TV as they were even ten years ago. Another shows that the more sexy shows a teen watches, the more likely she is at risk of getting pregnant. Then there's music, movies, videos, and social networking sites—not to mention the fact that it just takes one click of the mouse for someone to e-mail a naked picture of you to a thousand of your closest friends.

On top of all that social pressure, there's this physical fact of life. Not only are girls dressing older and acting older but their bodies actually *are* older, in some ways, than they used to be. Just a decade or so ago doctors wouldn't have expected your breasts to start developing until age ten. Now we know that your breasts might start budding as early as age seven or eight.[2] Meanwhile, if you're white, you're likely to get your first period about three months earlier than girls did forty years ago, and if you're black, it will come a good five to six months earlier than it did in the late 1960s. And two centuries ago girls hit puberty a good four or more *years* later than they do now.

We don't really understand all the reasons for the shift, but we do know that better nutrition and general health play a big role.

So with all this added pressure on you, are you getting lots of new information and new resources to help you deal with it all? Or a new level of respect for handling stress that previous generations just didn't face? Yeah, right. In your dreams.

That's why I wrote the book. A new kind of teen—that's you—needs a new kind of doctor. That's me.

R-E-S-P-E-C-T

The way health, sex, and physical information is handled by schools, teachers, doctors, and even some parents, you'd think today's girls were living in a time warp. Sex ed is still taught *exactly* the way it was thirty years ago (often it's all-abstinence-all-the-time). Most parents still have a tough time talking with their daughters about their bodies: Many parents don't even know the right words for the female anatomy. (Not that I blame them—their parents *never* talked to them about their bodies.) Even *doctors* don't seem to want to talk straight with girls. Old-school doctors always seem to fall into two groups: the "Just-Say-No" group (as in "Can we talk about safe sex?" "No.") and the "Free Love" group ("Whatever you do is beautiful. Just use condoms.").

Come on, people! This is the information age!

If you ask me, *both* these approaches are disrespectful to girls. I believe in giving you all the information you need, at the right age, so you can make smart choices for your body and your emotional health. That *doesn't* mean I'd tell you it's OK to have sex at a young age: In fact, I'll tell you all the medical reasons why that's not a good idea. But I'll also expect you to use your own best judgment and I'll treat you accordingly, with respect for the choices you make.

To make those choices, you need the very latest research and information presented in a straight-up way. That's why I wrote this book. I'm not going to take sides or preach one school of thought over another. You're smart. You know how to get information and you know how to think. I'm going to give you the right information at the right time and let you make the choices that are right for you.

LESSONS FROM THE RUNWAY

If there's one thing *Project Runway* has taught us, it's that one size or style does *not* fit all. I trust you. And I know you can make the decisions that fit you—your physical and emotional development.

To help you do that, I'm giving you all the facts, in a straight-as-an-arrow way, about pretty much everything your body will encounter through your teens and early twenties. In Section One you'll read about what to expect from your body in puberty—how to deal with period problems, infections, injuries, and hormonal issues. You'll also learn how to care for your breasts and bones for the rest of your life. In Section Two I'll give you the latest research and thinking on sex—what it means medically for your body, brain, and emotional health when you decide to hook up or have sex at early and later ages. I'll also explain the very strong medical evidence suggesting you should wait until at least eighteen for sex. Meanwhile, I'll tell you exactly how to protect and take care of yourself whenever you do make your decision about becoming sexually active. Finally, in Section Three, I'll tell you how to build a body that will last for the rest of your life—through healthy eating, risk control, exercise, and learning to handle mood problems.

To sum it all up, I'm basically offering you a free virtual visit to my office. I can't meet you and show you around like my actual patients. But I do want to welcome you to your new body and teach you everything you need to know to take care of it, love it, and enjoy it. I want you to own your body, because only you can care for it.

WANT A LATTE?

"Care for a chai? Some herbal tea? A latte?" my receptionist asks new patients when they arrive. They find her sitting at her glass desk in front of a curved wooden wall in the reception area of my office.

The beverage menu and the reception area are usually a surprise for new patients like Casey. "It looks like a spa," Casey told me. There's no big white counter or glass window to check in at. No ugly institutional gray carpet. Everything's done in cream, chocolate, and pale blue, with splashy red end tables and softly glowing wall sconces instead of the usual harsh office lights.

If you were a new patient, my receptionist would serve you your beverage of choice and snap a digital photo for your record—I like to "see" my patients when I'm reviewing their records or talking to them on the phone. Then, beverage in hand, you and, if you wanted, your parents would be escorted to my office, where you'd find fresh flowers on my desk. Later, if you needed an exam, you could slip into a comfy spa robe (not one of those flimsy paper or polyester gowns) in the exam room and watch TV on a plasma screen, check your e-mail on a Mac, or make calls while waiting for me.

And by the way, did I mention that everything's eco-friendly? I want to respect the planet, too.

The robes and the TV may all sound a bit much. It's not that I'm all New-Agey or that I'm trying to be some kind of Beverly Hills doctor to the stars. The truth is, it was just really fun dreaming up an office my patients would like. I mean, *nobody* rolls out the red carpet for teen girls, treating them like young women who deserve to be pampered and cared for. Only later, after we'd designed the new office and opened for business, did I realize just how much all the little details would mean to my patients. The details practically shout "I care about you. I want you to have a nice experience here. I want everything you see, hear, and touch while you're here to be respectful, soothing, caring."

After all, you have enough stress in your life. I should be helping ease it, not making it worse.

DOCTORS ARE A GIRL'S BEST FRIEND

OK, so not every doctor's office is going to offer you a latte. I'm not telling you to pick your doctor based on her taste in end tables. But I do want you to find a doctor who makes you feel respected, well cared for, and, yes, maybe even a little pampered.

That's especially important these days, now that girls are seeing gynecologists at a younger age. The American College of Obstetricians and Gynecologists—the huge national association that looks at data and makes recommendations for doctors like me—says that you should start seeing a gynecologist in your early teens, specifically between ages thirteen and fifteen. That's a surprise to most parents—especially moms, who probably didn't see a gynecologist until their senior year of high school or later.

If you're between thirteen and fifteen and haven't seen a gynecologist, you should (see the box on pages 13–15 on how to talk your parents into it). At the very least you need to see a gynecologist before you start having sex, so you understand all the medical consequences of your choices. For a lot of medical reasons I'll explain later, I think it's a really good idea for you to wait until you're at least eighteen to have sex. But if you decide to become active before that, it's my job to help you handle it in a smart way.

PRIVATES PRACTICE: MORE THAN JUST VAGINAS

Before they meet me, most of my patients think they're coming to see a "vagina doctor." But actually, "gynecologist" means the study of women—in my case, young women in particular. It's my job to be familiar with every health issue that might affect you as a member of the female sex. Sure, I can tell you if that funny bump or itch down there is something to worry about. (And, by the way, I don't want you *ever* to be embarrassed to bring stuff like that up. I have the same parts as you, and I do this all day long. To me examining a vagina is like examining an ear or nose—no big deal.) But I can also help you learn how to take care of your breasts, your bones, your weight, and your mental state—not to mention treating period problems and hormonal imbalances. My job as a gynecologist specializing in young women is to take care of the whole package and help you understand this new body you got when you reached puberty. Isn't that cool? I love my job.

It makes me sad that many girls never get to see a gynecologist until they're leaving for college—that's like studying for the SATs *after* you've taken the test. It's so much better to learn everything you need to know in your early teens, before you start running into the challenges you'll face

 DR. ASHTON'S PLAYLISTS

Over the years I've found myself repeating the same things over . . . and over . . . and over . . . to all my patients. These are things I really want them to remember, so I say them again and again. Sort of my personal playlist of advice. I've gathered up these lists and put them in boxes throughout the book, stressing the things I really want you to remember. Forgive me if I repeat information you've already heard, but these really are my greatest hits. Here are a few I share with my new patients:

- A new kind of teen needs a new kind of doctor.
- I respect my patients and care about their experiences—both in their lives and in my office.
- I don't take sides: I give my patients all the information so they (and their parents) can make good decisions. It's not my job to make choices for you.

? TRUE OR FALSE?

You should go see a gynecologist for the first time when you're between ages thirteen and fifteen.

TRUE.

You need both a pediatrician and a gynecologist when you're in junior high and high school.

TRUE.

You always need a pelvic exam when you go to the gynecologist.

FALSE. You don't usually need a pelvic exam unless you're sexually active.

later. Plus, a gynecologist like me probably will be the one doctor you see more of than any other medical profession later in life. The sooner you find someone you trust and can confide in, the better.

HOW TO TALK TO YOUR DOCTOR

Jessica and her mother first came to see me about a year ago. Jessica was thirteen, a flute player with a friendly face and short, glossy dark hair. Later I learned she had a radiant smile, too . . . but she definitely wasn't smiling when I walked into my office. She and her mother were sitting rigidly in front of my desk, waiting to talk to me about Jessica's painful cramps. They both looked like they'd rather be having their teeth drilled by a student dentist with a jackhammer.

I didn't take it personally. I'm used to being the only person in the room who isn't nervous on a first visit. Typically new patients like Jessica worry they'll have to put their feet up in the stirrups for a pelvic exam. Their parents worry that they're giving their daughter a green light for sex just by mentioning the *word* "gynecologist"—let alone taking her for a visit.

"So what's going on?" I asked.

I listened to Jessica describe her cramps, with her mom adding a few details now and then.

"OK," I said. "I think I can help. And don't worry—I don't need to do a pelvic exam."

"Really?" asked Jessica. I could almost see her white knuckles unclench. "You don't have to use that metal thing?" She meant the speculum, the instrument used in pelvic exams to gently open the vagina.

"Nope," I said. "We won't need that until you're twenty-one, or until you're sexually active—which I hope won't be until you're at least eighteen." I explained that very strong medical evidence suggests that it's much healthier to postpone sex as long as possible. From the corner of my eye I could see her mother relax. A few minutes later we were all laughing and chatting. BFFs!

Not bad, I thought. Five minutes into the visit, they both feel better. And we haven't even stepped in the exam room yet!

I just love my job.

Here are a few more things I tell all my new patients to help them feel a little better about the process. Understanding what to expect from your first visit can make your job and your gynecologist's job a lot easier.

1. You shouldn't be embarrassed.

All I do, every day, is take care of girls and women. We've all got the same parts. I've given birth, I've delivered babies, and I look at female anatomy *all day long*. To me looking at a vagina is *so* not a big deal. In fact, I'd rather look at a vagina than a foot (sometimes vaginas are *much* cleaner than feet!). If you take away just one thing from this book, remember this: Please don't ever feel embarrassed or ashamed of your body. Go ahead. Ask your doctor anything. She (or he) wants to help you but can't unless you say what's on your mind.

2. Anything you tell me is confidential.

By law I'm not allowed to tell your parents if you're sexually active or not. They can pound on my door and beg and plead, stalk me with phone calls or spam me online, and I'm still not going to tell them whether or not you're having sex.

There are only two conditions where I do have to break patient confidentiality:

- If I feel your safety or someone else's safety is at risk, I need to tell your parents and I might need to report my concerns to the appropriate agency or authority.
- If you have chlamydia or gonorrhea, the lab that processes the tests will *automatically* report it to the state health department. Your name will go on file as someone who has that particular STD, so the department of health can keep track of who gets what and make sure that everyone who needs treatment gets it. (Most of my patients find this rather alarming—and one more good reason to wait until at least eighteen before becoming sexually active.)

3. I trust you—but I'm not a psychic.

I expect that you'll be honest with me about what you're doing or not doing so I can treat you appropriately. If you tell me you're a virgin, I'm going to believe you . . . and I won't give you the same treatment as a girl who's sexually active. And if you don't tell me about problems you're having—itching, burning, discharge, whatever—I won't be able to help you.

Bottom line: If you're not honest with me, you won't receive the right medical treatment, and I won't be able to help you stay healthy. So don't be shy: Tell me what you're up to.

4. I don't need to do Pap smears or pelvic exams until you're sexually active.

That's a huge relief for most of my patients. But once you've had vaginal intercourse, you need to let me know—then it's time for what my patient Jessica called "that metal thing" (the speculum). As long as you're a virgin, I probably won't need you to put your feet in the stirrups. Most of my patients find this another very good reason to hang on to their virginity as long as possible.

5. Exams won't hurt.

One last thing to keep in mind. When you do finally need the stirrups and the speculum during your exam, please trust me that if the exam is done correctly, it really shouldn't hurt.

AN M.D. OF YOUR OWN

Many parents and girls don't realize that teens need both a pediatrician and a gynecologist. The pediatrician helps with health issues affecting kids of both genders. The gynecologist advises on issues specific to girls' growing bodies. Of course, good pediatricians know all about girls' issues, too, and can even perform pelvic exams. But—and of course I'm biased!—I think gynecologists like me, with specialized experience, offer girls special expertise and knowledge that only come from seeing patients like you all day, every day.

Unfortunately, many parents don't take their daughters to the gynecologist until the girls are about to leave for college. By then their daughters have missed the chance to learn about their bodies from an early age and to get important information and advice when they need it—like what you can do in your early teens to protect your breasts and bones for the rest of your life and how to make great decisions about sex. I don't blame parents: Many just don't want to think about the fact that your body is maturing, so it doesn't occur to them that you now also need a doctor who treats grown-ups, not just a pediatrician.

If you don't have a gynecologist of your own by the time you're in your mid-teens, talk to your parents about finding one. This might be a little awkward, especially if *you* think *they'll* think you're asking because you're sexually active (BTW, if you are, it's *even more important* to find a gynecologist soon). Here are three strategies to persuade your mother or father to help you find a great gynecologist when you're in your mid-teens . . . and hopefully long before you need one.

STRATEGY 1. Show your parents this book. Say "Mom (or Dad), the doctor who wrote this thinks it's a great idea to wait as long as possible for sex." (Your parents will really like that.) Then add, "I'd love to see a doctor like her. Can we find one?" You might also mention that adolescent gynos are not just "vagina" docs: We're the physicians who know the most about breast problems, bone health, period problems, and hormonal issues. What more could your parents ask for?

STRATEGY 2. Blame the cramps. If you have menstrual cramps, this is a great—and not too embarrassing—reason for seeing a gynecologist. This is the twenty-first century, after all, and suffering is *out*. Say "Mom (or Dad), these cramps are really bad and my friend So-and-So saw a gynecologist for hers, and it really helped. Can I do that?"

> **STRATEGY 3.** Ask your pediatrician. If you already have a doctor you see regularly, mention that you heard it's a good idea to see a gynecologist before you're sexually active, and ask if he or she can recommend one to you and your parents.

SURVIVOR—OR THRIVER?

When Jessica left the office after that meeting, she felt like she'd crossed a major milestone: She'd survived her first gynecologist's visit. And she was right—it *is* a big deal. She'd taken a crucial first step toward becoming a strong, powerful young woman who could keep herself healthy for the rest of her life. I know she felt a lot better after our visit. I'm hoping that as you read the rest of this book, you will, too.

Some days it seems like a miracle anybody makes it to adulthood. I mean, when I was a little kid, nobody even used seat belts, let alone car safety seats for babies and children! Airbags didn't exist, either. And I never even *saw* a bike helmet until college. I shudder to think of my own daughter (now nine) doing some of the things I tried in high school. Plus, she'll face all those new challenges that teens deal with today.

Still, I survived—and you will, too. But you know what? I want more than that for you. I don't want you just to *survive* your teen years. I want you to thrive. I want you to feel proud of your body, confident you can handle whatever it puts you through, and totally capable of making smart, well-informed choices. I'm lucky enough to know hundreds of girls who have done that, becoming healthy, confident, radiant young women along the way. And I know you will, too.

CHAPTER 2

EXTREME MAKEOVER

Puberty Edition

No matter how nice the spa robes in my office are, some patients are still pretty nervous when they come to see me for the first time. One new patient, fourteen-year-old Chelsea, came because her mother dragged her in to talk about her PMS symptoms. But when they arrived, Chelsea refused to talk to me at all! Instead she sat with her arms folded tightly across her chest, gazing sullenly past the roses on my desk and out the window beyond. She didn't even look at me. Her mother did all the talking. Later, in the exam room, Chelsea refused to get undressed so I could examine her. She and her mom ended up having a big fight right there!

I wanted to help Chelsea, but there's not much any doctor can do without even talking to—let alone examining—the patient. Chelsea ended up leaving in tears. A few hours later she calmed down and came back—this time ready to tell me about her symptoms and even let me take a look at her. Boy, was she surprised at how simple the exam was. I pressed gently on her belly and made sure she had the appropriate signs of puberty for her age—armpit and pubic hair and breast development. That was all. I didn't have to do a pelvic exam.

At the end she said to me with amazement, "That's it?"

"Yep," I said, "I promised you it wouldn't be bad."

Chelsea now comes to see me every six months—she's always on time, she never misses a date, and she tells me she actually looks forward to visiting.

I understand why Chelsea was so nervous during her first visit. Even though girls today are totally connected to a world of information, most adults aren't giving you nearly enough information about your own bodies. So when your body starts to go through the extreme makeover of puberty—changing from child to adult—some girls can get really freaked out. Some, like Chelsea, just want to block it out and pretend it's happening to somebody else's body. They've never been taught to care for their bodies the way they care for a new iPod or cell phone. They don't learn about all their body's nifty features or when to call technical support.

That's why Chelsea wouldn't talk to me at first. Until that moment when she decided to come back in, she never felt like she owned her own body.

Well, guess what? You *do* own your body. That's great news. But it's also a big responsibility. You need the right information. And you need a good help desk to call when it's not working right.

OWN YOUR BODY

Imagine the most embarrassing, personal health issue or the stupidest question you can think of. (Hideous bumps on your privates? Slimy ooze from sensitive places? A little fuzzy on the exact location of the vulva, vagina, and other parts south of the border?)

Now imagine you've got somebody you trust who's not at all embarrassed to answer your questions, who's utterly impossible to shock or gross out, and who knows how to solve your problem. That's me—and my fellow gynecologists who specialize in treating teens. Believe me, we've seen it all—from clitoral piercing (I removed one for a patient who couldn't get it out on her own) to wall-to-wall genital warts to every type of vaginal discharge. (BTW, if you're a virgin and the ooze isn't green, itchy, or smelly, it's probably nothing to worry about.)

In Chelsea's case it wasn't so much physical health issues like discharge that made her nervous. She—and her mom—just weren't used to talking about their bodies. Ever. Chelsea had never even heard of periods until she read Judy Blume at age ten. Later her mom gave her a pamphlet about menstruation and said, "Let me know if you have any questions."

This kind of well-intentioned silent treatment happens all the time. So many moms grew up not talking about their bodies with *their* moms that they don't always know how to talk with their daughters. It all seems like some deep, dark secret. Even if they *are* comfortable talking about body stuff, half the time (at least) their daughters—my patients—are so embarrassed that none of it sinks in anyway.

That's one reason why I wrote this book. Maybe—*maybe*—twenty or thirty years ago, the silent treatment was good enough. Maybe, once upon a time, "what you don't know won't hurt you" was actually true (although, frankly, I doubt it).

Not today. Like I said in chapter 1, this is the information age, people! How about a little—oh, I don't know—*information*, maybe?

You're growing up in a world that bombards you 24-7 with messages about your body, your weight, your clothes, and what you should or should not be doing with guys (or girls, for that matter). A world that tells you you're supposed to look sexy and act knowing and sophisticated. An age where three-year-olds wear underpants that say "Hot Stuff," where Paris Hilton first got famous because of (not in spite of!) a homemade sex video. Where somebody can post nude photos of you all over the Web in the time it takes you to read this sentence.

In today's world ignorance is *not* bliss and what you don't know *can* hurt you. If you're growing up today, you need to own your body in a way older generations never did. You need to understand it and know what's good for it and know how to take care of it from the moment it starts growing up. Love it or hate it (mostly love it, I hope), your body shouldn't be a big mystery. Make friends with it. Get to know it. Take it out for a movie now and then.

YOU'RE NOT A MINI-ME

Unfortunately, a lot of parents and teachers fall into what I call the "mini-me" fallacy. Even though they can see that teen life is totally different now than it was twenty or thirty years ago, they make the following assumption: "I was a teenager and I survived. You are a teenager, and therefore you will also survive." I've seen a lot of moms assume that their daughters' teenage experiences will be more or less identical to their own. I've also seen a lot of mothers assume that their daughters' teenage bodies are just small versions of adult female bodies. Like Mini-Me in the second *Austin Powers* movie.

But, actually, the bodies, minds, and emotions of tweens and teen girls are different from those of adult women in subtle but very important ways.

In this chapter I'm going to give you a tour of the extreme makeover your body will go through during junior high and high school and tell you exactly what you need to do to take ownership of your body—now and for the rest of your life. First, I'll help you understand the biological changes. Then I'll offer some practical advice on all kinds of stuff, from shaving and waxing to washing and taking care of your whole body.

Even if you've already gone through some of this, don't skip this chapter. It may help you understand where you've been and where you're going. And it will definitely help you answer that all-important teenage question, "Am I normal?"

ADOLESCENCE AND PUBERTY: KNOW MORE, STRESS LESS

Let's face it: "Adolescence" and "puberty" are funny, awkward-sounding words for times when bodies do funny, awkward things—like shooting up height-wise, sprouting hair in private places, and generating all sorts of odd and, shall we say, *interesting* new smells. Some girls just want to block this entire period out completely—the less said, the better. But, actually, it's a lot less stressful if you know what to expect. Here's the 411:

Puberty is the time when your body physically changes from child to woman. The first signs usually appear around ages eight to ten, but this ranges like crazy: Occasionally girls show the first signs of puberty as early as five or six! While puberty definitely doesn't run on a timetable, a typical schedule of events might look like this:

- Around age nine: Growth spurt
- Around age eight to thirteen: Breasts develop
- Around age ten to eleven: Pubic hair starts growing
- Around age twelve to thirteen: Periods usually start
- Around thirteen to eighteen: The brain matures, developing emotional and social intelligence, good judgment, and independence

As I said, this is *not* a train schedule. Each body is different. You'll have your own unique schedule of events.

Puberty is just a small part of the longer stage of adolescence, which ranges from your preteen growth spurt all the way through the end of high school and the beginning of college. Although your body *physically* reaches early adulthood by the mid-teens, you keep maturing emotionally and socially into your early twenties. During this time you might start dating or cozying up with someone you like. Most important, you'll start to develop the emotional maturity, common sense, and confidence you'll need to leave home and start life on your own (I know, it seems like that'll never happen—but, trust me, it will, sooner than you think).

Extreme Makeover: Puberty Edition

Ever wanted to be on a reality show? You're in luck. During your tweens and teens, your body's going to give you a mandatory makeover. Here's your before and after shot.

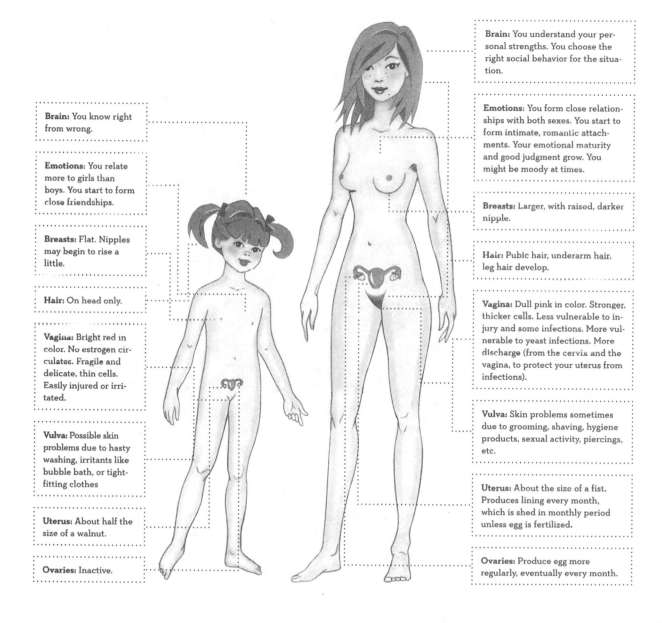

Brain: You know right from wrong.

Emotions: You relate more to girls than boys. You start to form close friendships.

Breasts: Flat. Nipples may begin to rise a little.

Hair: On head only.

Vagina: Bright red in color. No estrogen circulates. Fragile and delicate, thin cells. Easily injured or irritated.

Vulva: Possible skin problems due to hasty washing, irritants like bubble bath, or tight-fitting clothes

Uterus: About half the size of a walnut.

Ovaries: Inactive.

Brain: You understand your personal strengths. You choose the right social behavior for the situation.

Emotions: You form close relationships with both sexes. You start to form intimate, romantic attachments. Your emotional maturity and good judgment grow. You might be moody at times.

Breasts: Larger, with raised, darker nipple.

Hair: Pubic hair, underarm hair, leg hair develop.

Vagina: Dull pink in color. Stronger, thicker cells. Less vulnerable to injury and some infections. More vulnerable to yeast infections. More discharge (from the cervix and the vagina, to protect your uterus from infections).

Vulva: Skin problems sometimes due to grooming, shaving, hygiene products, sexual activity, piercings, etc.

Uterus: About the size of a fist. Produces lining every month, which is shed in monthly period unless egg is fertilized.

Ovaries: Produce egg more regularly, eventually every month.

- *If you're not sexually active, you usually don't need a pelvic exam at the first gyno visit.*
- *Teens are not mini-women: You might have the same body parts as an adult woman, but you're different in some subtle, and some not so subtle, ways.*

WHAT'S THE DIFFERENCE BETWEEN A VULVA AND A VAGINA?

"Um, Dr. Ashton . . . I'm not quite sure which is the vulva and which is the vagina," my patient Lynn confessed.

I get questions like this all the time, and love them. It's your body! Learn about it! For some reason our society seems very shy (or sly?) about using the right terms for the female body. You'd be surprised how many times I get calls from other doctors saying a patient has a problem "down there." If *doctors* can't even bring themselves to use the right terms, it's no surprise that many girls and women aren't sure what's what!

I don't care what pet names you give your anatomy—I have one patient who calls her vulva "Larry"—but I do want you to at least know the proper terms so if you ever have a problem, you can easily describe it to a doctor (who probably isn't acquainted with "Larry"). Plus, knowing and using the right words helps give you a sense of ownership over your body.

Oh—and the answer to Lynn's question: The vagina's inside, the vulva's outside. Although a lot of people use the term "vagina" to refer to all the female genitals, technically the vagina is just the tube leading from the cervix to outside your body. The vulva is the external area of your genital region—basically everything you can see outside and inside the outer lips (or labia majora—the lips with hair). In addition to the labia majora and minora (the inner lips, without hair), the vulva includes the opening to the vagina, some tiny glands, and the clitoris—a little tiny mound of "erectile tissue," which, like a nipple or a penis, fills up with blood and gets firm when aroused.

DID YOU KNOW?
A Five-Year-Old Monkey Is More Grown Up Than a Human Teenager

Humans have the longest puberty and adolescence of all primates. For humans in the United States and other Western cultures, "puberty" (when your body physically changes from a biological child to a young adult) lasts almost eight years, compared with a couple of years for rhesus monkeys, who reach adulthood by age four or so. For humans, adolescence is a very long period that includes important emotional and social development. Typically this period happens between ages ten and the early college years. It may even last a lifetime. Ever met a grown-up who still acts like a teenager? These folks definitely take the idea of "forever young" a little too far.

HOW OLD IS SHE, REALLY?

When I was watching the 2008 Olympics with my kids, we got into a big debate over the real age of the gold medal winner in gymnastics, He Kexin of China. She just didn't look old enough to compete in the Olympics. You have to be sixteen, but she looked more like twelve. The rest of the world argued over it, too. It was impossible to tell her age because, like many teen gymnasts, she looked like a young girl. Later that fall investigators determined she really was sixteen. She kept her gold medals.

It turns out that super-strenuous exercise like Olympic training can delay puberty, including the start of periods. So can malnutrition, anorexia, or other eating disorders and chronic disease like kidney failure or cancer.

We don't truly understand why puberty comes late for these girls. But we *do* know that you need a certain amount of body fat for puberty to begin. I'm not talking about *being* fat, I'm talking about *having* fat—a healthy layer of body fat, the kind that doesn't make you look big. Super-athletes just don't have that healthy fat.

Among other functions, body fat produces estrogen and other substances important for puberty. This link between body fat and puberty makes perfect biological sense. Your body figures no fat means there's not enough food available. "Oh, no!" it thinks. "There must a famine! This would be a bad time to start a family!" So, no fat, no puberty; no puberty, no babies. Smart body, huh?

REMODELING: MEET YOUR NEW BODY

During puberty and adolescence, you basically move into a new body—the one you'll live in for the rest of your life. Treat it well and you'll have a palace to enjoy for decades. Get to know it, get to love it, and learn to take care of it. Here's a quick tour of the new you. But, first, meet the crew making all these changes.

The Star of the Show: Estrogen

Bigger breasts, a grown-up reproductive system, monthly periods—none of it would happen without estrogen. This hormone affects just about every change your body will go through in puberty. Estrogen's sort of like the host on *Extreme Makeover: Home Edition*. Sure, there's a house with a lot of rooms there—ovaries, uterus, fallopian tubes—but not much happens till the host kicks off the show. Suddenly the painters are painting, the carpenters are hammering, and everything snaps into high gear.

Most of the estrogen in your body is produced by your ovaries, two small structures in your pelvis that produce eggs as well as hormones. But fat tissue produces some estrogen, too. No one knows exactly what triggers the production of estrogen in puberty, but once it starts pumping, your whole body changes. Before the estrogen arrives, your bones get longer and you get taller in a growth spurt around age nine. Later—a few years after your first period—estrogen helps close the growth plates in long bones like the legs, so you don't keep getting taller and taller for the rest of your life (see chapter 5 for details). Your ovaries start releasing eggs. Your uterus grows a monthly lining and sheds it. So it's no wonder if you feel especially moody or irritable as you go through puberty. It's not easy living in a place where every room is under renovation.

❓ TRUE OR FALSE?

Girls Have Estrogen Instead of Testosterone, and Guys Have Testosterone Instead of Estrogen

FALSE. Both have some of each. Everybody has some testosterone. In teenagers it's produced largely in the adrenal glands—where adrenaline is made—which are located on top of the kidneys. These glands also produce two more hormones that are similar to testosterone. And guess what—testosterone is also produced by the ovaries (confusing, huh?). All this testosterone produces body-hair growth in both gals and guys. Meanwhile, guys also have some estrogen, too, produced by body fat, which plays a role in their growth.

JOB DESCRIPTION: ESTROGEN

If you want something done right, you have to do it yourself. Estrogen gets involved in pretty much every event of female puberty. Major entries in its job description include:

Developing breasts
Slowing height growth
Accelerating metabolism
Reducing muscle mass
Increasing good cholesterol and lowering bad cholesterol
Slowing bowel functions
Increasing blood-clotting factors (so your body can stop bleeding
    more easily once your period starts)

WHAT'S NOT NORMAL?

There's such a wide range of normal that sometimes it's easier to tell what's *not* normal. If you're reading this book, your body's probably already passed through some of these stages, but the whole list gives you an idea of just how different bodies can be.

- If pubic or armpit hair starts growing before age seven or eight, girls should see a doctor and get a special blood test that checks for abnormal production of testosterone. (Yep, testosterone—the male hormone. We all have it. See the box on the top left.)
- Girls whose breasts start developing before age seven (for white girls) or six (for African-American girls, who sometimes develop earlier) need to see a doctor. Most of these girls—75 percent, in fact—are just (very) early bloomers who won't need any treatment. But some will need monthly shots to make sure their early flow of estrogen doesn't prevent them from reaching their full height.

DR. ASHTON'S PUBERTY PLAYLIST

- A vulva is not a vagina. The vulva is on the outside, and the vagina's on the inside. (If you remember this, you'll know a lot more than most women do!)
- Puberty is different from adolescence. Puberty is a physical thing and adolescence is the whole long period of emotional and physical change that happens throughout your teens.
- There's a big range of "normal" when it comes to puberty.

Upstairs Renovations: Budding Breasts

Your puberty makeover starts upstairs. Breasts develop in stages starting around age nine. Doctors call these "Tanner stages," but you can think of the stages as:

- **Raisins:** There is a slight raising of the nipple (around age nine to ten).
- **Buds:** Small mounds of tissue form behind the nipple (around age ten to eleven).
- **Swelling:** The buds swell, but there's still no clear difference between the breast and the nipple.
- **Nipples:** A secondary mound forms where the nipple (or areola) is clearly separate from the breast (sort of like a cherry on top of a scoop of ice cream).
- **Mature breasts:** They reach their full size, usually in your late teens.

I'll tell you everything you ever wanted to know and more about your breasts and how to treat them in chapter 5. For now, here are some of the main concerns I hear from my patients:

One breast is bigger than the other! Yep, this happens sometimes. Usually they even out over time. Occasionally they don't. One sixteen-year-old patient I had ended up with one B-cup and one A-cup breast. It bothered her so much she decided to have plastic surgery to even them out. But don't worry—that's usually not necessary.

My breasts aren't growing! Chances are, that's perfectly normal. If your mom was a late breast bloomer, you might be, too. And if you're super-skinny, don't expect big things in the boob department, since you won't have much fat tissue to develop into breasts. Don't give up hope, though: Breasts continue to grow and change as late as age twenty-five! If you're concerned about your breast size, don't be shy—ask your doctor about it. Remember: It's *always* better to ask and stop worrying, no matter how embarrassing the question, than to live with needless anxiety.

There's a bump under my nipple! Sometimes a small, semihard bump forms under the nipple. This can be pretty scary for girls and their parents. Most of the time it's just a rapidly growing breast bud. But see a doctor about it if it's still there after a few weeks, if it grows quickly, or if it hurts.

There are hairs or little bumps on my nipple! Nothing to worry about—just a normal part of some maturing breasts. Some young women pluck the hairs or have laser hair removal.

My breasts hurt! I really am sorry to tell you this, but it's perfectly normal for your breasts to feel sore, especially right around the time of your period. This happens because the breasts respond to changes in your body's levels of hormones. Try Motrin, cutting back on caffeine, or sleeping in a sports bra.

RED FLAGS: BREAST HEALTH

If you have either of these two symptoms, please tell your parents and go see a doctor ASAP. There may be nothing to worry about, but you need a doctor to check them out.

NIPPLE DISCHARGE. It's *not* normal for any liquid to come out of the center of the nipple. If you see any liquid (which might be white, green, or reddish-brown) from your nipple, go see a doctor.

ROUND LUMPS. Anything that feels like a marble, a pea, or a grape—hard and round—could be a benign breast cyst. These small lumps can occur due to normal changes in breast tissue, infection, injury, or some medications. If you feel something like this, flip to chapter 6, where I talk about these issues. You'll want to see a doctor soon.

Downstairs Renovation: All Vaginas Are Not Created Equal

As I'm fond of telling my patients, a vagina is not a vagina is not a vagina. Unlike, say, elbows or knees, which all look and behave pretty similarly, every vagina has its own disposition. Some are pretty hardy and rarely troubled by a yeast infection or an itch or a smell. Others are much more sensitive: Take one mild little antibiotic for a sinus infection and, whammo!— the yeasties check in . . . and they don't check out. That's because for some women, taking antibiotics kills off the "good" bacteria that normally live in the vagina, letting the "bad" bacteria—or yeast—run wild and cause an infection.

To make matters worse, just when you think you've got your vagina figured out, it changes. Your private parts will be very different at ages eight, eighteen, and fifty-eight. Here's an overview of the transition you'll go through during your tweens and teens.

Your Vagina Changes. As your body starts making more estrogen during puberty, it changes the cells in your vagina. They become paler in color, so your vagina no longer looks bright red on the inside. The cells also become stronger. This is great news, because they're less sensitive and less susceptible to injury. Meanwhile, the vagina gets longer, reaching about four to six inches in length on average. Fortunately, the vagina's on the inside, not the outside (the outside part is the vulva), so you won't even notice.

Your Cervix Changes. Meanwhile, your cervix gets busy doing its job: keeping unwanted intruders—specifically bacteria—out of your uterus. The cervix is a donutlike opening at the end of the vagina, deep inside your body. Like a bouncer at a hot nightclub, it's supposed to keep out everyone but the most exclusive of visitors. Only sperm are welcome at this party (if and when you're ready for babies, that is!). One of the main ways the cervix keeps out bacteria is to produce mucus, which catches and expels unwanted intruders, so they don't make their way into your uterus, your fallopian tubes, and the rest of your body.

Your Mucus Changes. If you start seeing more white, clear, or yellowish gloppy stuff in your underwear, it doesn't necessarily mean you've picked up something nasty. It's just your cervix working overtime. It's making mucus, guarding you from infection and keeping you healthy. Although you may not love it, remember (and say this with me): *The presence of mucus in the vagina is totally normal.* If it's not green, smelly, or itchy, chances are good (especially if you're a virgin) that there's no problem. I'll describe the few exceptions in chapter 4.

Your Period Starts. Meanwhile, your uterus starts doing its job, too. It produces a thick lining, called the endometrium, whose job is to nurture fertilized eggs. Of course, unless you're pregnant, there *aren't* any fertilized eggs to nurture, so the endometrium gets tossed out once a month along with the blood that nourishes it. When this happens, you get your period. (Doctors call the onset of your first period "menarche," BTW.) Some girls find it annoying to bleed once a month. Others take it as a badge of womanhood. A lot of girls feel both ways at the same time.

Either way, it's a pretty cool process from a scientific point of view. The uterus is one of the only examples of the human body repeatedly destroying and repairing cells. Pretty sexy stuff if you're a biologist.

With your first several periods, your ovaries usually haven't started releasing eggs yet. Eventually they'll release an egg every month, but that probably won't happen consistently for six to eighteen months after your first period. For some girls ovulation doesn't occur regularly for up to five years after their first period. This means your periods might not come predictably or last the same number of days for a long time after you start menstruating.

DID YOU KNOW?
Girls Were Younger in the Old Days

If you've heard your parents say that ten-year-olds now seem a lot older than when your parents were kids, they're actually right. It's not just because girls have cell phones at age eight, either. Physically, girls really do develop sooner now. As I mentioned in chapter 1, periods start a few months earlier than they did forty years ago, but breasts develop a few years earlier. And in the United States periods start about four years earlier than they did for girls two centuries ago. One reason is that most girls in the United States eat better and are healthier than in the past. Good nutrition and good health tend to bring on periods earlier. Also, patients and doctors are more attuned to subtle signs of puberty and development, so they can recognize puberty and acknowledge its presence more quickly now than folks of previous generations did.

? TRUE OR FALSE?

Vitamins Can Help Keep Your Vagina Happy

TRUE! New research has shown that vitamin D can help reduce irritation in your vagina, by keeping your immune system healthy and your skin surfaces happy. I usually recommend that my teenage patients take a supplement of 1000 units of vitamin D3 a day.

- Leave the vagina alone! Don't put creams, lotions, potions, soap, or other liquids in the vagina unless a doctor tells you to.
- The job of the cervix is to make mucus: The vagina should be moist. If it were dry, you'd be in menopause (and about fifty years old).
- Not every bump in your pubic area is a sexually transmitted disease. But if you're sexually active, have it checked by a doctor, just in case.

GO WITH THE FLOW: SOME POINTS ON PERIODS

We'll talk a lot more about periods in the next chapter. But here are some highlights. If your bleeding patterns are noticeably different from what I describe here, please read chapter 3 carefully and see a doctor soon.

- Your cycles may not be regular for six to eighteen months after your first period, but by the end of that time you should be able to predict when your period will start.
- Most "regular" periods happen every twenty-four to thirty-six days. But some girls have cycles as short as twenty-one days or as long as forty days.
- Your cycles should be about the same number of days each month, not twenty-one days one month, forty the next, and thirty-six the next.
- The average period lasts three to seven days.
- Normal periods do *not* include passing large clots of blood on a regular basis.

When I refer to the length of your menstrual cycle, I mean the time between the first day of your period in one month and the first day of your period in the next month. So if you got your period on September 1 and October 1, that cycle was thirty days. And day fifteen of your cycle would be fifteen days after your last period started.

FAMILY FEUDS: BALANCING YOUR BACTERIA

As your vagina makeover nears completion, all sorts of visitors drop by to take a look. Some move in uninvited. We're talking bacteria here. Every vagina has lots of it, all different types. Like relatives, some are good, others not so much. Usually they coexist peacefully without major family blowouts. But now and then one branch of the family gets unruly and tries to take over. The result is usually itching, burning, discharge, odor . . . and a very unhappy person attached to that vagina.

One common uprising is called bacterial vaginosis (BV), usually caused by the overgrowth of a bacteria called *Gardnerella*. When these bacteria run amok, they produce a great deal of thin, grayish, discharge, with a nasty, fishy odor. Although BV is not technically a sexually transmitted infection, unprotected sex can trigger it. But even virgins get it sometimes. If you notice your underwear smells like something out of *Finding Nemo*, see a doctor. It's annoying, but antibiotics clear it up.

Another family feud breaks out when candida—or yeast—overpowers the good bacteria in your vagina. There are lots of kinds of yeast—the most common is called *Candida albicans*—and all of it can cause itching, discomfort, and discharge. To treat it you apply a cream or take a pill; we'll discuss treatments in the next chapter.

For now just remember this: The best way to keep peace in your privates is to *leave the vagina alone!* The less you put in it, the better. Don't put in creams, medicines, or anything else unless a doctor tells you to.

 DID YOU KNOW?
You Can't Get Yeast Infections Until You're in Puberty

If you already had doubts about the joys of puberty, here's one more drawback: yeast infections. If you had itching, burning, uncomfortable vaginal infections as a child, you might have been told, or concluded from TV commercials, that you had yeast infections. Nope. Turns out young girls usually can't get vaginal yeast infections until they have estrogen circulating in their systems. Estrogen provides the right environment for yeast to flourish. So little girls, who don't yet have estrogen in their bodies, don't get yeast infections. But once you're in puberty, your body puts out the welcome mat for the yeastie beasties. If you have any uncomfortable itching and burning, you might have a yeast infection. Don't just buy something over the counter for it: Go see a doctor.

PRIVATES PRACTICE: DOS AND DON'TS

Here are more good practices for your privates.

Do: Go bare at bedtime. Sleeping without undies gives your bikini region a chance to air out, which can help prevent infection.

Do: Wipe from front to back. This keeps bacteria from spreading from your rectum to your vulva and vagina.

Do: Wear cotton underwear—it breathes better.

Do: Wash the vulva, vagina, and all its folds, nooks, and crannies gently, with baby shampoo or gentle soap.

Do: Pat the vulva dry with a clean towel after bathing—don't rub.

Don't: Scrub the vulva.

Don't: Linger in a soapy bath. A long soak in soapy water can cause itching and irritation to your vagina and vulva. If you like long baths, skip the bubbles.

Don't: Use perfumed products in your bikini region.

Don't: Hang around in a bathing suit, sweaty underwear, or gym clothes for long periods of time. Bacteria and yeast love moisture.

Don't: Use feminine hygiene products like creams or douches (products that rinse the vagina with chemicals that supposedly clean it—but really do more harm than good).

HAIR EVERYWHERE

At the same time you get your new and improved body, you'll start noticing a few other changes. Hair is one of the most obvious. Pubic hair, which usually first appears around age eleven but sometimes even earlier, starts out as sparse, lightly colored hair at the top of the vulva or pubic bone. By the late teens it gets darker and curlier and spreads over the pubic bone in a triangle and down over the labia.

How much body hair you have depends on your age and ethnic background—but also on what's in style. Back in the 1960s (or so my mom tells me) a lot of women chose not to shave their legs and underarms. Today, on the other hand, we're in a "less-is-more" phase: My fellow gynecologists and pediatrician pals sometimes joke that nowadays you can't tell if a patient's hit puberty just by checking for pubic hair . . . because the second it develops, many girls remove it.

Our American obsession with body hair removal sometimes leads to funny situations. Like the time my friend, who's a doctor, was getting dressed with her five-year-old daughter in the room. Her little girl knew that women had hair on their genitals—but she *didn't* realize they had armpit hair. Apparently my friend needed a shave that day. As she took off her PJ shirt, her daughter shrieked, "Mommy! You're growing vaginas under your arms!"

My friend's daughter may have been a little unclear on her anatomy, but she was right about the similarity between pubic and underarm hair. The hair follicles in those areas respond to testosterone, which makes them twist and kink—so your pubic and underarm hair is curlier and coarser than the hair on your head. Fortunately, hair in those areas also stays shorter than hair on your head.

A HAIRY SITUATION?

Some women experience a condition called hirsutism, which means excessive body hair. This may include hair on your inner upper thighs that spreads down the legs; a lot of coarse hairs extending from your pubic triangle to the belly button; or on your chin, neck, or sides of your face, or between your breasts. Sometimes excessive hair indicates a hormonal imbalance that needs treatment. If you think you have a lot of body hair—even if everyone else in your family does, too—you should ask a doctor about it.

If you do have excessive hair, two types of medication can help. One is the good old birth control pill (yes, it helps with hair control, too!). The other is a medication called Spironolactone. These medications reduce the amount of testosterone floating around in your blood. Both usually take at least six months to start working, so you won't see a difference for a while.

HAIR CARE DOWN THERE

It was 5:50 a.m. on a Thursday when my beeper went off. The screen flashed the name of one of my patients, Michelle. Usually when I get a page there's also text describing the problem. This time the screen was oddly blank, except for Michelle's name and phone number.

When I called her back, her mother answered. "Dr. Ashton, we're so sorry to bother you so early, but . . . well . . . um . . . let me put Michelle on to talk to you herself. . . ."

Puzzled, I waited a few seconds while Michelle took the phone. She told me that while trimming her pubic hair on the occasion of her sixteenth birthday, she had cut her labia with the scissors. Ouch.

"Are you bleeding?" I asked. She was. And she was scared: A flap of skin was hanging off and she was afraid she might need stitches. I told her to meet me at the emergency room.

Fortunately, when I examined Michelle, I found the cut wasn't serious. I cleaned it out and applied some antibiotic ointment. I was relieved, Michelle was incredibly embarrassed, and her mother was in a state of complete shock. Talk about a birthday surprise.

REMOVING HAIR SAFELY— DOS AND DON'TS

A slip of the scissors doesn't happen often, thank goodness. But removing body hair from your bikini region, legs, or underarms can cause other problems. The most common is an infection called folliculitis, which causes ugly little bumps and can really ruin a nice bikini line.

Here's some advice for avoiding your own birthday surprise.

SHAVING. Personally, I love using my husband's shaving cream. He doesn't love it so much, trust me. Neither will your brother, if you have one, so I recommend getting your own shaving cream. And it is an absolute medical *must* that you get your own razor. Sharing razors is a serious medical no-no:

Razors can pass infections from one person to another via microscopic cuts or nicks of the skin, resulting in tiny amounts of blood landing on that razor blade. So don't use your bro's razor, your mom's razor, or your BFF's razor. Get your own. Believe me, you don't want a skin infection—or, even worse, a blood infection.

Do: Shave in the same direction that the hair is growing. This is hard to do for the legs but easier for pubic hair, which grows down, toward your feet: Shave in that direction—this will reduce the chances of getting folliculitis.

Do: Use a clean, sharp, new blade whenever you shave.

Do: Apply a shaving cream or gel to the area before running a razor over it (I know this *sounds* obvious, but we've all done stupid things in a rush to get to the pool).

Do: Shave in the shower or bath, where your skin's already slick and wet.

Do: Shave after you've washed your skin well. Bacteria love little ports of entry into your skin, where they can sneak in and throw a big infection party. Use soap first, then shave.

WAXING. Waxing sometimes strikes me as some sort of primitive rite of passage. Applying hot wax to various hairy parts of the body, and then ripping it off with shredded cloth? Can you believe we actually pay for this?

Well, *I* pay for it, anyway. After all, it's safe, fast, and effective for almost every part of your body, from your upper lip to your arms, legs, and pubic region. I actually talked my brother, a plastic surgeon, into waxing his back—once. He said I should have given him a bullet to bite on. At least he learned to appreciate what we women suffer through for beauty's sake.

He could have had it a whole lot worse. True fact: When I was sixteen I went for a bikini wax, and the inexperienced beautician left the wax on too long. She couldn't get it off after she'd placed the little strip of cloth over it. She wound up pulling and tugging so hard that I wound up with a giant bruise/blood clot/blister right on my bikini line! I thought my poor mother was going to have a heart attack. Here are a few ways to avoid a nightmare like this:

Do: Go to a professional salon where they really know what they're doing. Take it from me—you do *not* want someone practicing on you with hot wax.

Do: Make sure the salon uses clean wax for each person. If they dip a tongue depressor into the wax to apply it to your body, ask them to use a clean one for you.

Do: Ask them to do small areas at a time rather than bigger regions of hair. Even though the overall process takes longer this way, it will actually be easier and safer.

Do: Take Motrin or Advil before your appointment to reduce pain, redness, and swelling. Use icepacks immediately afterward.

Don't: Have any waxing done twenty-four hours before a big event. Trust me: You will *not* look your best!

LASER HAIR REMOVAL. Basically, a laser directs very high powered light energy at the base of the hair follicle and damages it. The good news is that it's very effective, although most of the time it doesn't eliminate hair growth entirely. The bad news: It's uncomfortable and not cheap, costing upward of several hundred dollars. It's also time-consuming and usually takes several sessions.

If you go this route, find someone who's highly trained at laser hair removal. You don't want anyone practicing on you with a laser! Good cosmetic dermatologists, plastic surgeons, and even some gynecologists are usually the people to trust. Also, remember that some skin colors and some hair types and colors respond better to laser treatment than others. So do your research before you hand over your parent's credit card.

ELECTROLYSIS. A hair-thin metal probe is inserted into the hair follicle itself and then charged with a light electrical current to destroy the hair follicle forever. Not as popular as laser hair removal—but it's technically the only way to permanently remove hair. Be sure to do your homework as to the costs, risks, benefits, and time involved.

GRUESOME GROOMING GAFFES

So what if you do end up with a birthday surprise or other grooming issue? Here's what to do for the two most common problems:

If you cut yourself, expect a lot of blood. There's a generous blood supply to the pubic area, so cuts bleed *a lot*. Fortunately, all that blood also promotes quick healing. Apply firm direct pressure for ten minutes. Don't stop to take a peek at how your cut is doing—that could start the bleeding again. The pressure should be about the same as a firm handshake; anything stronger could bruise your skin and make you even more sore later. If after ten minutes you're still bleeding, or the cut seems really bad, tell your parents or go to the doctor. Like Michelle, you probably won't need stitches, but better safe than sorry.

Nasty-looking little bumps: If you find pimply little bumps in your bikini area, you may have folliculitis, which happens when the bacteria that's normally all over our skin enters a small nick or gets into the hair follicle itself. The resulting infection looks like a big pimple. The shaving advice above will help you avoid this. But if these suckers still appear, ask your doctor to prescribe an antibiotic lotion. I often prescribe one called Clindamycin and tell my patients to put it on the shaved or waxed area twice a day for two to three days, starting the day they remove the hair. This usually clears the problem up quickly.

THE SKINNY ON SKIN

No chapter on the joys of puberty would be complete without facing up to your face. What teen doesn't know the agony of the gigantic pimple that rears its ugly head at the most humiliating time? A whopping 85 percent of teens have acne, the medical term for pimples, zits, craters, honkers, or undergrounders, so it's the rare teen who *doesn't* have firsthand experience with this condition. But don't despair. There's a lot you can do to prevent and treat acne.

Anatomy of a Zit

What causes zits? Each and every pimple is really nothing more complicated than a tiny skin infection. Each little infection causes a halo of redness and sometimes pus in one small area of your face or body (which doesn't feel small *at all* if it's *your* face or body). Hormones, sweat, skin-to-skin contact, and even certain medications can play a role in acne. And skin problems often run in families, so knowing if your parents or older siblings had acne can help you plan ahead in waging your war on zits.

Here's how it works. Think of acne as a cast of four characters: First there's bacteria—which is perfectly normal and covers your skin all the time but which sometimes invades your oil glands and causes an infection. Then there's the oil itself produced by the glands, which you need to keep your skin from drying out and cracking like ice. Then there are pores—the little entrances to the oil glands—which sometimes get clogged when there's an infection. And there's inflammation—the redness, swelling, and sometimes pus that builds up around the tiny clogged pore as your body tries to fight off the infection.

Having just one of these four factors—bacteria, oil, clogged pores, or inflammation—can cause a zit. But when several factors are out of balance, forget it. It's a veritable nonstop pimple party.

"Aha!" you say. So all we need to do is decrease oil production or bacteria. Then the pores won't get clogged or inflamed. If only it were that simple, you and I would both be millionaires with our surefire acne cure.

But here's the catch. Every single person is different from a medical perspective, and your acne is caused by your own particular body chemistry, the environment, and your skin's own unique personality. For some teens zits result from too much oil production. For others particularly nasty bacteria play a greater role. So there's no "one-size-zits-all" solution (ha!).

Of course, that's not what you'll think if you cruise the aisles of the drugstore. Stop in the skin-care section, and you might easily conclude that everyone with acne has it for the same exact reason, and all you need to do is buy this or that product. Problem solved.

But the truth is a lot more complicated. In order to stage your best attack on acne, you need to understand the root cause of your particular case. Often a skin doctor, aka dermatologist, is your best hope. But a thorough pediatrician or gynecologist can certainly help, too.

Zit Zappers: Acne Treatments

Usually a skin doctor will start by prescribing something that you can apply to the surface of your skin, known as a topical treatment. This may be an antibiotic (to target the bacteria) or something with benzoyl peroxide (which helps dry out the oily parts as well as wipe out bacteria).

If these two topical treatments don't work, your doctor might prescribe an antibiotic pill to try to cut down on the aggressive bacteria. Unfortunately, the bacteria that cause zits are often resistant to a lot of antibiotics, so zits can be trickier to treat than, say, strep throat. In these difficult cases we bring out the "big guns": the class of drugs known as retinoids. Accutane is one well-known type of retinoid. I took it myself when I was twenty-two, and, actually, it was pretty tough. It's a very powerful medication that's not that much fun to be on. It can make your skin very sensitive, which might make it feel like the zit situation is actually getting worse (although it's not). Among its other nasty side effects, it can cause severe birth defects, so dermatologists are required by law to make sure girls taking Accutane are also on birth control.

The flip side of Accutane is that it's extremely successful at clearing up zits permanently. Once the zit-causing bacteria is completely gone from your skin, it's unlikely to come back. However, if you'd rather go more natural, some studies suggest that diluted tea tree oil applied with a Q-tip directly to your zit can help reduce bacteria. You can find this on the vitamin aisle in a natural food store.

Just remember, no matter how bad your acne is, most cases can be treated very effectively. Just promise me that you won't let bad skin get to you; almost everyone goes through it and knows exactly how it feels to have a breakout. Don't let that cause a breakdown.

ALERT: ZITS ON THE BACK AND CHEST AREN'T COMMON

Even though 85 percent of teens deal with acne, it's not common for girls to have pimples on the back or chest. If you have zits there regularly, it may be a sign of a common hormonal imbalance. Check with your doctor.

ZAPPING THE ZITS: COMMON ACNE TREATMENTS

Antibiotic gels or pills

Benzoyl peroxide

Retinoids like Accutane

Natural therapies like tea tree oil diluted and applied with a Q-tip
   to the zit

DOES SOMETHING SMELL FUNNY IN HERE? HANDLING INTERESTING ODORS

Babies smell great (most of the time). Teens, on the other hand, develop more interesting grown-up smells. Why?

One reason is sweat glands, located all over your body, responding to all kinds of stimuli, from exercise and the weather to stress and illness. Sweat itself doesn't usually smell bad. But when sweat meets the bacteria that lives on your skin, and it's all mixed up together in a dark moist place (like your armpits), or, better yet, somewhere with hair (like your privates), it creates quite a bouquet. Just be glad you weren't born before the Golden Age of Deodorant.

For girls the vagina—and the mucus made by the cervix—offers another source of smells. Normally mucus shouldn't smell bad. But it might if you have an infection like BV, which I mentioned on page 34.

To Keep B.O. on the Down-Low:

Do: Shower daily.

Do: Use a mild, gentle soap—or, even better, mild shampoo—to clean your entire body.

Do: Clean in between all folds of skin.

Do: Wash from head to toe, not toe to head. If you use a washcloth, wash your face *before* your privates.

Never: Douche or put soap or liquids inside the vagina. This disrupts the delicate bacterial balance in the vagina and can cause annoying problems.

Never: Use talc powder around the crotch. Some studies have linked excessive powder around the genitals to an increased risk of ovarian cancer.

"AM I NORMAL?"

Remember Chelsea, my terrified patient at the beginning of this chapter? Like so many of my patients, she turned out to be a quick learner. Before long she became totally comfortable talking to me about her periods and pretty much everything else. "I love knowing that I can ask you *anything*," she told me.

I love it, too. I know she's getting the info she needs to take charge of her own health for the rest of her life. That's what I want for you, too.

CHAPTER 3

PERIODS

Your Questions and Exclamations

L ori had always been a great student at her all-girls school. Then came tenth grade. Suddenly the cramps that had always come with her period got much worse. Every month pain shot up her back and down her legs, making it hard to walk or even sit. She started missing two or three days of school every month and her grades dropped. Friends teased her for being a wimp. They had no idea she was throwing up from the pain.

Finally she came to see me.

"I've tried everything," she told me. She sat fully clothed on the exam table and I sat on my favorite rolling stool. "Advil, aspirin. I even tried these PMS pills I found at the drug-store."

"Yeah, I've seen those," I said. "They don't work."

"They were a total rip-off," she admitted ruefully. Then she asked, "Am I just being a whiner about this? I mean, everybody gets cramps, right?"

"Not like this," I said. "I've been there. It know how miserable it is."

Back in high school my own cramps were almost as bad as Lori's. We're talking rolling-on-the-floor, curling-up-in-a-ball-crying cramps. My mother—a nurse, mind you—thought this was a bummer, but perfectly normal. She had bad cramps, too. "That's how it is," she told me.

But that's not true anymore. "You don't have to live with period pain," I told Lori. "This is the twenty-first century. Suffering is *out*."

I explained to Lori what exactly causes period pain and other menstrual symptoms and what her options were. In this chapter I'll tell you the same things.

A LOVE/HATE RELATIONSHIP?

My nine-year-old daughter, Chloë, recently asked me if "people can tell" when a girl first gets her period. I thought that was a pretty sharp question for a third-grader.

"Nope," I answered. "You don't look any different. But you might see yourself differently. Maybe a little more of a grown-up, less of a kid."

A lot of my patients enjoy that added sense of maturity and find it exciting to get their first period. But it doesn't take long before many of them develop a love-hate relationship with their periods. On the one hand, expecting your period and appreciating its regularity can teach you about your body's rhythms and give you a sense of control over your health. That's the love.

Then there's the hate. Although it's probably not really hate—it's more like fear, anxiety, or worry. Before your period starts, or during the first few times you get it, you might worry you'll bleed to death (you won't) or that your tampons or pads will leak or smell funny (they won't if you change them often), that you won't be able to do the same things as usual (with very few exceptions, you will), or that people will be able to tell you have your period (they won't). Once your period is regular, you may have another set of worries altogether. Monthly cramps, headaches, and moodiness, anyone? Not to mention inconvenience and the constant low-level worry. If it comes, you're miserable. If it doesn't, you worry. How can you win?

IS THIS NORMAL?

The "hate" part is even worse if, like Lori or me, your period always comes with cramps, nausea, or a host of other miserable side effects. To make matters worse, still today some moms, teachers, and even doctors just don't realize how bad the pain can be—or that severe period symptoms aren't normal, and can and *should* be helped.

One lesson I learned from my own terrible cramps was that just because something's common—as cramps were, in my family—doesn't mean it's normal (that is, something that almost all bodies do and are supposed to do). I think it's a great idea to talk to your family and friends about your health, your body, and your experiences and to ask them about theirs. But you also need a reality check from an actual doctor about what's normal. In med school they make us take exams on this stuff.

Plus, if there's one thing I've learned from my patients, it's this: For teen girls and periods, it's hard to know what a "normal" period really is. Periods are very irregular in the early years, and every girl's body is different. There's never one "normal"—say, cramps or no cramps. There's always a range—as in, it's normal to have some cramping but not normal to roll on the floor and miss school.

Sometimes you can even be outside the normal range and still have no medical problem. For instance, at age fifteen my patient Carrie had very irregular periods—her cycle might be four weeks in June, six weeks in July, and five weeks in August. She'd asked her friends and her mom about it, and none of them had such erratic cycles. So when she came to see me, she already knew her body wasn't in the normal range. By the time you've had your period for a few years, cycles are usually the same length from month to month. I ran some tests, expecting to find that Carrie had a hormonal imbalance—but she didn't. There was nothing physically or hormonally wrong with her. Her irregularity most likely was just her body's own quirk.

The moral of the story is that "normal" is a range. In this chapter I'll give you some information to help you figure out if you're in that range. If you fall outside it, you should see a doctor. Maybe nothing's wrong and you'll feel very relieved. Or maybe there's an easy treatment for a problem that's been bothering you. And, of course, in the unlikely event that something's really wrong, the sooner you know, the sooner you and your doctor can find a solution.

NORMALITY CHECK

While nobody but a doctor can tell you if your body is normal or not, it's a great idea to talk to your family and close friends about their health experiences. It helps you understand your own health and helps you feel more open about talking about your body. Here are some questions you can ask your girlfriends and family.

Sometimes when I have my period, I feel [bloated, depressed, like eating everything in sight, etc.]. How about you?
How often do you get your period and how long does it last? [Every month, like clockwork? More often or less? Five days? Seven days?] Do you get [headaches, nausea, fed up with never having tampons when you need them]?

Some people will tell you every month and that it lasts up to seven days. Others may say "whenever." The more people you ask, the more you'll see what a range of bodies and experiences there are when it comes to periods.

This happens to me [I go through a box of tampons a day; I can't stop eating chocolate; I snap my brother's head off, etc.]; does it happen to other people, too?

WHY WE GET PERIODS:
THE CLIFFSNOTES VERSION

My patient Jolie had heard it all in health class and even from her mother. But she still wasn't totally clear on why we get periods. So I gave her the CliffsNotes version.

1. At puberty the brain starts sending chemical signals to your body, via estrogen and other hormones, saying it's time to get down to the work of reproducing.

2. Those hormones wake up your ovaries and uterus. You reach menarche—your first period. After that your brain sends chemical signals out roughly once a month, telling your body to get ready for a baby. Every month powerful hormones, including estrogen and progesterone (another important reproductive hormone), rise and fall in your system.

3. For the first two weeks of your monthly cycle, your uterus builds up a nice cushy lining to nurture a fertilized egg. Estrogen and progesterone are both necessary to build up the lining. I tell my patients they can think of estrogen as the building blocks of the endometrium and progesterone as the cement that holds it all together. You usually need both, in balance, for a healthy reproductive cycle.

4. In weeks two and three of your cycle, estrogen reaches its highest levels.

5. In weeks three and four, the ovaries crank up progesterone production. Around week three (or more precisely, usually two weeks before you get a period), the ovaries release the egg. The timing of this egg release is very unpredictable in teens, so it's basically impossible to time when you're fertile or not fertile. That's why the "timing" method of birth control does *not* work for teens.

6. In week four, if the egg isn't fertilized, the uterine lining is flushed out and you get your period.

7. Repeat from Step 1.

Yep. In the days before birth control people died sooner, and women spent a lot of their lives pregnant and breast-feeding (both keep you from getting your period). A baby girl born in the United States today will probably get her period around age twelve, have two children, and possibly breast-feed for six to nine months each. Let's say that means three years when she's not getting her period. Then around fifty-one she'll hit menopause and her periods will stop. That adds up to about 36 years of periods—or roughly 468 periods during her life. (And you thought this was a health book, not a math text.)

But a girl born in 1900 probably would start her period later, have more children, breast-feed them for longer, and live until about age forty-eight. She might only have periods for about twenty-five years total, or about three hundred periods. Imagine the money she would have saved on tampons if they'd existed back then.

WHERE'S YOUR SPOT ON THE RANGE?

Before you look at the chart below, repeat after me: "Normal is a range. Being outside the range doesn't mean there's a problem—but I should see a doctor."

NORMAL	NOT NORMAL
Bleeding lasts 1 to 7 days.	Bleeding lasts longer than 7 days.
Cycles (the time between Day 1 of one period and Day 1 of the next) last about 21 to 40 days. The middle range is 28 to 30 days, or every 4 weeks.	Cycles last less than 21 days or more than 40.
Cycles are usually the same from month to month. (Say, 21 days, or 30 days, or 35 days every month.)	Cycles jump around in length—21 days one month, 30 days the next, 40 days after that, etc. Even though these cycles are all in the normal range, it's *not* normal to vary so much.
Advil or Motrin help your cramps.	Your periods are so painful that you miss school/come home early on a regular basis.
You soak a pad or tampon in several hours (although you may change it more often).	You soak a pad (so no white surface shows at all) in 1 hour or less. You bleed so heavily that you routinely stain your clothes.

PERIOD PROBLEMS

It's a rare woman who gets through her life without a cramp, pain, or other period problem. Cramps, aches, irregular bleeding, and other menstrual issues are the top reasons that new teenage patients come to see me.

I tell them that most period problems start with hormones, which affect your whole body, not just your ovaries and uterus. They're linked to everything from your skin to your appetite. They also seem to affect brain chemicals called neurotransmitters, which affect your moods. Since so many period problems are caused by hormones, many can be treated with hormones, too—specifically the birth control pill.

But there are lots of other ways to treat period problems, including heat therapy, healthy eating, meditation, and other methods. I'll tell you about all of them so you—working with your doctor and your parents—can make the choice that's best for your body.

Surprise! Expecting the Unexpected

"Um . . . does anyone have a tampon?"

My patient Jaida was running for sophomore class president. Twenty minutes before her big speech, she found herself in the girls' room, begging anybody who came in for sanitary supplies. Although she'd had her period since age twelve, she still hadn't settled into a predictable pattern and was always getting surprised. Fortunately, a girlfriend with a well-stocked purse rescued her in the nick of time. Jaida (who won the election) visited my office the following week.

I determined there wasn't anything wrong with her physically and she didn't really need treatment. But I encouraged her to start a "period diary," something I think all my patients should do. She followed my directions below for several months and found that although her bleeding was still irregular, she could predict within a ten-day window when her period would come—and she made sure she always stocked her purse with tampons during that time.

Dear Diary . . .

You don't need a lock and key for a period diary—just a regular wall calendar (which you don't need to keep in the kitchen). I recommend doing this for at least six months, but many women always track their periods. On your calendar, note:

1. **The days your period starts and ends.** Make an X on the first day of bleeding and keep making Xs every day until you stop bleeding.

2. **The severity of cramps or other symptoms.** Use a scale of 0 to 5 (0 = no problems, 5 = your worst symptoms) to describe how intense the symptoms are on each day. For instance, your cramps might hit Level 4 on Day 1 of your period but subside to 2 or 3 on the next two days, and then go back to zero. After six months,

look back over your calendar and see if you can find any patterns. Just knowing that your cramps will only last a day or two can make you feel better.

3. **How much you bleed.** This one's a little tricky. Most medical texts say the normal amount of bleeding is about five tablespoons and one teaspoon per period. But how in the world would you measure that? Walk around with a measuring spoon in your underwear? An easier way is to estimate how long it takes to completely soak a pad or tampon to the point there's no white surface showing. If it takes less than one hour, that's not normal, and you should see a doctor. Of course, my patients often change their pads or tampons before they're completely soaked through, so I just tell them to note how often they change them and how soaked they are (is a pad 50 percent white? 75 percent white?). You don't have to be super-precise about it: The point is to have an overall record, so you notice if there's a month when you're suddenly bleeding much more or less than usual.

If you keep your chart for several years, you might notice that your bleeding gets lighter as you age (yay!). Bleeding tends to be heavier in the first few years of your period. That's because at first your ovaries aren't always releasing eggs every single month. A cycle without an egg (which is called anovulation) is usually heavier and sometimes lasts longer than cycles with an egg. The good news is, anovulation usually goes away as you mature, so the bleeding gets lighter and shorter.

Occasionally anovulation and the heavy periods it produces come from a hormonal imbalance. These are usually easy to treat: You can read all about them in chapter 5. In any case, keeping a period diary will help you and your doctor figure out what's going on with your body.

PAINFUL PERIODS

Not a day goes by when a patient doesn't come in for help with cramps, aches, and other period-related pain. That's not surprising. Studies show that 60[3] to 92[4] percent of teenage girls have painful periods. So if you're dealing with pain, know you're not alone. About 15 percent of girls have pain that interferes with their daily lives, sometimes to the point of missing school or activities.[5] Another 15 percent of teens have pain that's not bad enough to send them to the doctor—but does send them to the pharmacy, looking for over-the-counter solutions. Only fourteen out of one hundred teens with painful periods ever seek help for their problem.[6] And one out of three parents whose daughters had painful periods was unaware that their daughters were suffering.[7] (As a mom, this last part really breaks my heart!)

Painful periods (which doctors call dysmenorrhea) usually result from one of two problems:

1. "The Bullhorn Problem." These are pains and other symptoms caused by normal physical and hormonal processes in your body (that's what was happening with Lori). Your body's sending the right signals but sending them a little too loudly—and causing side effects like cramps, headaches, moodiness, or other symptoms. It's like your body's using an electric bullhorn instead of a cell phone to talk to your ovaries.

2. "The Plumbing Problem." Less often period pain can be caused by a physical problem with the pelvis, like an injury, infection, or abnormal growth in the uterus. In other words, it's a problem with the physical "plumbing." For example, I treated one thirteen-year-old patient in the emergency room for pain so severe she was throwing up. The ER doctors thought she had appendicitis, but CT scans showed a rare physical condition. She essentially had two cervixes, with a wall dividing one side of her uterus and vagina from the other! One of her cervixes was blocked, which caused a buildup of blood that didn't flow out with the rest of her period. Two simple operations cured the problem. Her condition was rare, but other, more common physical problems can also create this kind of problem (which doctors call secondary dysmenorrhea).

℞ DR. ASHTON'S PERIOD PLAYLIST

- You don't have to live with terrible cramps. This is the twenty-first century: We believe in treating pain.
- No "specially formulated for PMS or periods" remedy sold over the counter actually works. Don't buy them.
- Oral hormones—aka "the pill"—are a very common treatment for period pain. Most concerns about the pill are based on myths. For the most part the pill can be a safe and effective therapy for many period-related problems, including cramps.

? TRUE OR FALSE?

Everyone Gets PMS

FALSE. Technically, premenstrual syndrome *only* affects about 40 percent of women.[8] If that sounds low, it's because PMS is technically defined as a "diagnosable" medical condition with symptoms that are so severe they interfere with your life—keeping you home from school or away from activities, say, and in serious discomfort. Some women also suffer from premenstrual dysphoric disorder (PMDD), which brings severe depression or mood disorders with it.

But even though most women don't officially have PMS, teens may be more likely to have it than adult women, with an estimated 14 to 88 percent of teens having moderate to severe symptoms, like cramps, irritability, headaches, food cravings, bloating, depression, or anger.[9]

QUIZ: NORMAL/NOT NORMAL

Which of these period symptoms are normal?

A. Mild cramps that ease up when you take two Advil or Motrin
B. Cramps that not only don't respond to Advil but actually make you cry
C. Moodiness or irritability
D. Food cravings
E. Weight gain of one to two pounds
F. Mild headaches
G. Severe headaches or headaches that interfere with your vision

H. Tiredness

I. Lack of concentration

J. Mild sadness or lack of interest in your favorite activities

K. Depression: Unstoppable crying jags or persistent dark thoughts

L. You miss school or skip activities for a day or more every month

M. Acne gets worse

ANSWER. B, G, K, and L are *not* normal. If you have these symptoms, see a doctor. The others are all typical symptoms women experience before their periods.

SUFFERING IS *OUT*: WHAT YOU CAN DO

From the quiz above, it should be pretty clear that even in normal periods, your monthly cycle can affect a lot more than your uterus and vagina. Some symptoms are easy to explain. Cramps, for instance, happen because your uterus contracts when it sheds its lining (called the endometrium)—similar to the way it contracts during labor. No wonder it hurts. It's like giving birth!

As for all those other symptoms, researchers don't have the ultimate answer. They do think that fluctuating hormone levels (specifically, estrogen and progesterone) and another compound called prostaglandin play a role in many types of menstrual misery—from zits to headaches to making your family wish you'd move out. Sometimes these symptoms get bad enough to qualify officially as PMS (see the box above), but usually they simply qualify as "severe" or "painful" periods. And there's a lot you can do for them.

I'll describe them here and then tell you about a wide range of things that can help. Your best bet is to see a doctor and try a range of treatments until you figure out what works best for your body.

Severe periods can occur every single month or just once in a while. They usually start within six to twelve months after your first period and may get gradually worse as the months go by, as they did with my patient Lori. The pain usually starts the day before your period comes or else a day or two after. My patients often describe the pain as coming in waves, affecting their lower abdomen or pelvis. Sometimes it radiates down their lower back or upper thighs. Some people also experience bad headaches.

None of these symptoms are fun. Fortunately, there's a lot you can do.

NORMAL OR NOT?

NORMAL MENSTRUAL SYMPTOMS
- Mild cramps or aches for a day or two
- Being a little tired, grouchy, or sad
- Being a little less interested in your favorite activities

NOT NORMAL: SEE A DOCTOR
- Extreme changes in your mood or behavior
- A headache you'd call "the worst headache of your life"
- Inability to eat or hold down food or drink
- A temperature over 101°F
- Lots of nausea, vomiting, diarrhea
- Abdominal pain that ibuprofen doesn't help
- Pain when you pee

TAKE TWO ADVIL AND CALL ME IN THE MORNING

Not so long ago menstrual symptoms were considered an inevitable part of life (at least by my mom). Welcome to the twenty-first century! Now medical science knows you don't have to live with pain and misery every month. You've got way too much to do. So see a doctor for severe symptoms that interfere with your daily life (see the box on page 59 for guidance on when to see a doctor). Meanwhile, here's a range of things that you can do yourself that might help.

Ibuprofen. The best way to treat period pain is with something doctors call nonsteroidal anti-inflammatory drugs (NSAIDs) but which most of us call Advil or Motrin—brand names for ibuprofen, a very common NSAID. (Sorry to keep using this ugly abbreviation, but there *are* other drugs in this class besides ibuprofen, and I want to be super-accurate.) Unlike other pain relievers, these go straight to the cause of the pain, targeting prostaglandin production in the uterus and counteracting its painful effects on the uterine muscles. Generally safe, these drugs don't make you sleepy, give you the jitters, or have other side effects. But don't take ibuprofen if you're allergic to aspirin—you might have a dangerous cross-reaction.

DOCTOR'S ORDERS: ADVIL OR IBUPROFEN FOR CRAMPS
- Start with **400 milligrams (2 pills of 200-milligram strength) every four hours** beginning on the day before you expect your period. Always take NSAIDs with food to protect your stomach.
- If that dose level doesn't work, **try taking 3 pills of 200 milligrams every six hours.**
- If that still doesn't work, ask your doctor for a stronger prescription-strength dose.

Note that Tylenol is not an NSAID and is not the best treatment for period pain.

COMPLEMENTARY TREATMENTS: NUTRITION, EXERCISE, HEAT, AND TOUCH

My patient Olivia had terrible cramps that started when she was about sixteen. When even prescription-strength ibuprofen didn't work, I suggested the other standard prescription for severe periods—oral hormones (aka birth control pills).

Olivia and her mother both looked a little nervous when I mentioned the pill. Even though it's perfectly safe and often used for period pain (I'll explain in depth below), they just weren't comfortable with it. Olivia's mother felt she was too young to be on the pill and Olivia herself wasn't crazy about the idea either.

"I totally understand," I told them both. I'd examined Olivia, and after she was dressed we all sat in the exam room. "There are lots of other remedies we can try." After all, women have been having period pain since way before birth control pills and ibuprofen were invented.

Some people call natural remedies "alternative therapies," but that makes it sound like you have to pick one or the other. Actually, with a few exceptions that I'll mention, you can try these *and* ibuprofen or other treatments. Since most of these treatments can work together, I prefer the term "complementary" therapies. Many of them have helped my patients. They're safe and usually easy to try yourself. And there's an added bonus: If they work for you, they might also help you with other problems later in life! For example, if meditation helps ease your period pain now, it might help with arthritis later on. So see what works for your body.

Healthy Eating. Some nutritionists believe that restricting certain foods, including dairy, sugar, salt, wheat, and caffeine, can help reduce menstrual pain. In fact, entire books describe food and eating plans that might help PMS and painful periods. Specifically, some nutritionists advise the following:

- Limit sugar, dairy, "empty carbs" like cookies, and white bread.
- Limit processed foods (anything that comes ready-made in a package, from fast-food burgers to breakfast cereal).
- Eat more whole grains, fruits, vegetables, and seeds.
- Drink a glass of blueberry, huckleberry, or other juice high in antioxidants and essential fatty acids daily (I really like acai berry juice, which has great anti-inflammatory properties).

While there's not much scientific evidence proving that food choices can reduce period pain, there's no doubt that sensible, healthy eating in general is good for you. So I recommend that all my patients give healthier eating a try.

"Even if it doesn't help your pain," I told Olivia, "it will promote overall good health for life." I added that a food strategy like this could also help her stay at her healthiest weight for life.

Exercise. "Yeah, right, gimme a break," you're probably thinking. "I can't even stand up straight on the first day of my period, and Dr. Ashton's telling me to put on my *running shoes?!?*" You're 100 percent right: Exercise is *not* a quick fix for period pain. But aerobic exercise—running, biking, swimming, anything that gets your heart pumping—produces natural substances called endorphins. These endorphins produce a mild physical euphoria (ever heard of the "runner's high"? Or notice how happy you are after soccer practice?). When you're in pain, these endorphins act like a healthy version of morphine—they help you relax and they take the edge off the pain.

I'm not telling you to go jogging when you're having bad cramps. But I *am* saying that a regular exercise routine incorporating thirty to forty-five minutes of aerobic exercise three to five times a week may help ease your symptoms over the long haul. I can't promise it will help. So far conclusive scientific evidence is lacking. But regular physical exercise also happens to be one of the single most powerful things you can do to stay fit for the rest of your life. So what have you got to lose?

Vitamins and Supplements. According to the latest research, some dietary supplements might help with period pain. You can find these at any good vitamin store. Specifically:

Magnesium. Lots of studies have shown that magnesium can help lower levels of a certain type of prostaglandin and ease period pain for some patients. I recommended that Olivia try 500 to 1000 milligrams of magnesium. *But* I also warned her not to take more, since magnesium can be dangerous in higher doses. If you try magnesium, take it starting on Day 15 of your cycle until your period stops. And take it in magnesium glycinate form (other forms might cause diarrhea, or loose poops). And never take more than 1000 milligrams per day.

Omega-3 Fatty Acid Supplements. I also suggested that Olivia might try an omega-3 fatty acid supplement—specifically, fish oil. One study showed that adolescents who took a fish oil supplement for two months had less period pain. But high doses of fish oil may also have high doses of vitamin E, which can cause heavy bleeding when combined with NSAIDs. So don't try omega-3 fatty acid supplements (or vitamin E supplements) *and* ibuprofen or similar NSAID drugs. It's either/or. If you try this, take 1 gram of omega-3 fatty acids per day, dividing it into four doses a day of 250 milligrams, and take it with food, since that helps you absorb it and helps keep your stomach from getting upset. Check the milligram amount on the label carefully before taking it—otherwise you won't know how much is in each dose.

DON'T TRY THESE AT HOME

Avoid any over-the-counter medication claiming to be specially formulated to reduce menstrual symptoms. These treatments simply don't work, so don't pay extra money for them. Just go get some Advil, try the techniques above, or see a doctor.

I also **do not** recommend herbal remedies reported to ease period symptoms, such as black cohosh, blue cohosh, and wild yam. **Do not try these.** Although they have powerful estrogenlike effects, they have not been well studied. In my opinion, the risks definitely outweigh possible benefits.

OTHER NO-NOS

Don't: Take vitamin E supplements, even though some studies suggest they might help. If you take even small doses of vitamin E while you're also taking ibuprofen or other drugs in the NSAID class, your risk of uncontrolled bleeds increases—including bleeds in the brain.

> **Don't:** Take high doses of magnesium (more than 1000 milligrams) unless directed by a doctor.
>
> **Don't:** Take omega-3 fatty acid supplements (fish oil) **while also** taking ibuprofen or similar NSAID drugs. That's because some fish oil supplements also contain high doses of vitamin E.

Heat Therapy. The good old-fashioned hot water bottle ain't just for Grandma. Reports of heat therapy for pain date as far back as the second century A.D. from as far away as China and India. Although there aren't a lot of modern medical studies on the topic, researchers think heat reduces menstrual pain by stimulating heat receptors that lie just beneath the skin. This may keep some types of nerve cells from sending pain signals to the brain. The heat also increases blood flow to your abdomen, which might dilute pain-causing compounds. And more blood flow brings more oxygen to the uterus, which could help, too.

DOCTOR'S ORDERS

To try heat therapy:

- Apply moderate heat to your lower abdomen for six to eight hours. To do that, use a hot water bottle, warm towel, or a newer device called ThermaCare, a heating pad that doesn't use electricity (it uses a chemical reaction to basically rust itself into a hot state). The pad remains hot for eight hours and you can wear it under your clothes, which is helpful if you're at school.
- Don't use an electric heating pad: It could cause a fire, and we don't fully understand the damage that electromagnetic fields may inflict on cells.

Massage and Therapeutic Touch. "Here we go again," you're thinking now. "When I'm having cramps, the *last* thing I want is for anybody to touch me." Still, some patients report that massage and a technique called therapeutic touch, developed in the early 1970s by a nurse at New York University, can help increase relaxation and reduce pain, or at least the perception of pain. Many doctors are skeptical about how effective these techniques are, because no rigorous scientific evidence supports it, but some patients swear by them.

To try these therapies: Locate massage or therapeutic touch practitioners specifically trained to ease period pain. To find reputable practitioners, ask around for recommendations. Some more progressive doctors' offices or insurance companies may be able to refer you.

Meditation, Hypnosis, and Guided Imagery. Studies say these relaxation techniques can reduce pain and suffering and speed recovery for open-heart surgery patients. If it helps with cardiac patients, it probably can't hurt with your cramps. These techniques involve taking yourself through mental and physical steps that help you relax and deal with pain. To try it, find a practitioner trained or certified in complementary or alternative medicine, or a certified practitioner of hypnosis. The American Society of Clinical Hypnosis has a list of certified hypnotherapists at www.asch.net. And many psychologists, therapists, and practitioners of alternative or complementary medicine are trained in these techniques. After a few sessions with an experienced practitioner, you'll be able to do this for yourself. Good news: If these techniques help you with your period pain, they may help you cope with other stressful or painful situations later in life.

Acupuncture. The ancient practice of Chinese acupuncture has been studied extensively in both Western and Eastern medicine. While we still don't fully understand why it may work, I tell my patients that acupuncture is safe and can be very effective therapy for painful periods. Best of all, the risk is very, very low. The worst that can happen is that it won't work. Many health care providers and even spas offer acupuncture services these days. Most states require acupuncture practitioners to be licensed. To find one near you, visit the American Academy of Medical Acupuncture at www.medicalacupuncture.org.

HAPPIER HORMONES: TREATING PERIOD PAIN WITH THE PILL

Thirteen-year-old Brooke came to see me for horrible cramps. High-dose Motrin cut her pain in half within a few months. I could have prescribed oral hormones, but I usually try to avoid prescribing hormones within two years of the first menstrual period, while systems are still "working out the kinks."

Two years later Brooke developed an unrelated problem—a benign ovarian cyst (see chapter 7)—which we treated with oral hormones to help prevent it from coming back. She didn't get any more cysts—and most of her period pain disappeared, too!

If you've tried other remedies and nothing helped, your doctor probably will talk to you about oral hormones—aka the birth control pill. Since most period pain is caused by hormones, regulating those hormones via the pill usually solves the problem. Oral hormones really work well. They reduce menstrual symptoms and make periods lighter, shorter, and less painful. Plus, they cut the risk of ovarian cysts and pelvic inflammatory disease and have lots of other benefits.

Oral hormones combine estrogen and progestin (a man-made form of progesterone) to prevent your body from releasing an egg every month. As long as you're taking a pill—often for three weeks every month—your body won't shed its uterine lining. When you take a few days off the pill (typically once a month), you get your period. But it's not a real period, since you didn't ovulate, and it's more controlled than a naturally occurring one—we call this a "pill period." After you're on the pill for a few months, your periods usually become shorter, lighter, less painful, and more regular. All this can really boost your sense of control and confidence.

When I prescribe oral hormones for period problems—especially for patients who are under eighteen and still virgins—I don't call them "birth control pills." I make a point of calling them "oral hormones," to drive home the idea that this is a treatment for a medical condition, not a prescription to go out and start having sex. As we'll talk about later, there are health advantages to holding off on sex until you're eighteen. When you do start having sex, you'll need to use *two* forms of birth control—not just the pill.

THE PILL: MYTHS AND FACTS

My patient Lori, the one I mentioned at the beginning of this chapter, wasn't having much luck with the prescription-strength NSAID drug or the complementary remedies she tried, so I suggested oral hormones. She hesitated.

"This'll sound dumb," she told me, "but I really don't want to gain weight."

"Don't worry, that's just a myth," I told her.

Lori's mother was nervous about the pill for a different reason—she was worried I was giving Lori a permission slip for sex. But when I explained the benefits and risks, Lori and her mom decided oral hormones were a good idea.

FAQ: TOP QUESTIONS ABOUT THE PILL

Will I gain weight? Unlikely. The pill has zero calories. Most people don't gain any weight on the pill. A few girls do gain one or two pounds, probably due to fluid retention. But it's not enough for anyone to notice. If you gain more than ten pounds, the culprit is probably not the medication but your eating habits or a hormonal situation.

Does the pill cause cancer? Many people think the pill has been linked to all kinds of cancers. Actually, oral hormones are one of the only ways to *reduce* your chances of developing ovarian and uterine cancer. In fact, a woman can reduce her risk of ovarian cancer by as much as 50 percent by taking the pill!

Isn't the pill linked with breast cancer? Lots of studies have been done to determine whether oral hormones increase or decrease breast cancer risk. The current consensus among most leading experts is that it does not *significantly* increase breast cancer development—but it may increase the rate of breast cancer *detection*.

What about cervical cancer? Cervical cancer is very rare. Oral hormones do seem to slightly increase your risk, but we don't understand why. In fact, it might be that women taking birth control pills may be less careful about always using condoms—and unprotected sex leads to a greater chance of getting HPV, which can lead to cervical cancer. But it's also possible that oral hormones change the cells of the cervix and make them more prone to HPV infections and subsequent cancer.

Bottom line: If you take oral hormones, have gotten the HPV vaccine, and—once you're no longer a virgin—always use condoms during sex, cervical cancer is not a significant risk, in my opinion.

Who shouldn't take the pill? There *is* one group of people who shouldn't take oral hormones: those with rare clotting disorders. The pill can increase the risk of blood clots in the leg, the lung, or the brain (a clot in the brain causes a stroke).

For most people these are very small risks. But if you have a close family member who had a blood clot in the leg (called a deep vein thrombosis) or the lung (a pulmonary embolism) or who had a stroke, or if your mother had a lot of miscarriages, you may be at higher risk. Your doctor can perform blood tests to see if you have a clotting disorder that would make the pill a bad idea for you.

People who get certain kinds of migraine headaches may also be at higher risk of stroke. I had one eighteen-year-old patient who came to me for help with period pain. I started her on a low-dose pill. Soon after, she was diagnosed with a rare form of migraine that can create visual problems lasting for days. I consulted with her pediatrician and her headache specialist, and we decided she shouldn't be on the pill. I prescribed high-dose ibuprofen instead.

Will the pill make me shorter? OK, this isn't really a frequently asked question, since most of my patients don't know about the pill's effects on bones. But it's pretty interesting, so I slipped it in here. Remember, in the last chapter I mentioned that estrogen plays a role in your growth? It helps you build strong bones. But, ironically, it also helps close the growth plates in your bones during your teens. So if you take oral hormones—which include estrogen—during the first year or two of your period, your growth plates may close earlier than they would otherwise, and you might not reach your full height. So instead of being 5 feet 6 inches, you might top off at 5 feet 5 1/2 inches. To avoid that I usually don't prescribe oral hormones for girls who've only recently started their periods. Still, some situations are so severe that oral hormones do make sense, even for girls who've only been menstruating for a year or two—but only for a brief period of time.

Overall, oral hormones are incredibly safe. If you're generally pretty healthy (aside from your period problems, that is), the risk of dying from taking an oral hormone is lower than that of dying in an automobile accident. You probably get in a car every day because you have a long way to go and the risks are small. Oral hormones are similar. For most girls with severe period problems, the big benefits outweigh the smaller risks.

 DID YOU KNOW?
The Pill Can Reduce Some Cancer Risks

Oral hormones are one of the *only ways to reduce your risks* of ovarian cancer. That may be because you don't ovulate when you're on the pill—and scientists think that one type of ovarian cancer happens at least partly because monthly ovulation damages the ovary's outer capsule. Multiple pregnancies and prolonged breast-feeding also prevent the ovaries from releasing eggs and seem to offer the same benefit.

Using oral hormones for a long time can also reduce uterine cancer. When the uterus is exposed to too much estrogen, without progesterone, it can cause abnormalities in the uterine lining, which can lead to cancer. Oral hormones reduce this risk by controlling the levels of progesterone and estrogen.

? FALSE OR FALSE?
Myth-Perceptions About the Pill

Here are a few common myths and misunderstandings about the pill.

You have to start on a Sunday.

FALSE. Your body has no idea what day of the week it is.

The pill causes weight gain.

FALSE. I've said this before, but it's worth repeating, since this is such a common concern. The pill has no calories. You might retain a little water, but if you gain more than two or three pounds, blame something else.

Taking the pill for a long time can make you infertile.

FALSE. Your body's own hormonal system kicks back in just a few days after you get off the pill. It has no affect on your future fertility.

> *You need to take a "break" from the pill now and then.*
>
> **FALSE**. There's no need to take a month or a year off the pill at any time.
>
> *You need to take one week off the pill every month.*
>
> **FALSE**. Actually, in some cases, and with some formulations of the pill, you don't need to take a week off in order to have a period. So you could go several months without having a period. There are no bad effects from controlling your cycle with the pill so that you skip periods altogether for several months.

NOT A LICENSE FOR SEX

Lori's mom told me privately that she was afraid that putting Lori on oral hormones would give her the green light for sex. I reassured her that's not the case.

"You know, fear of pregnancy actually isn't the major reason girls decide not to have sex. They wait or don't wait because of peer pressure, the values of their friends and family, concern about their reputation, or just plain good judgment. Being on the pill probably won't affect her decision one way or the other."

I also remind parents that this is a great time to revisit the "what you didn't learn in sex ed" discussion. Whenever I prescribe oral hormones for girls who are virgins, I tell them it's incredibly important to their future health to wait until at least eighteen to have sex—and even longer is better (see chapter 8). I also remind them that the pill doesn't prevent sexually transmitted diseases. (You should see their faces when I open my huge medical textbooks and show them actual photos of women with herpes, genital warts, syphilis, and pus-filled blisters. It makes quite an impression.)

And, of course, I remind them that even if they never, ever miss a single pill, one in one thousand women who take the pill will *still* get pregnant. Of course, most women and teens do miss a pill now and then: In that case, 8 percent of women will get pregnant on the pill. You heard me. That's eight out of one hundred. I've delivered several babies who were "pill accidents." I even know several women *doctors* who got pregnant this way. If it can happen to doctors, it can definitely happen to you.

 DID YOU KNOW?
You Can Get Pregnant on the Pill

Even when women take the pill faithfully, every single day, exactly as prescribed, one in one thousand still gets pregnant. And 80 percent of women *don't* take it perfectly—they miss a pill now and then. In this typical instance, eight in one hundred women will get pregnant while on the pill.

DON'T SUFFER, BE HAPPY

Eventually we got Lori on a regimen of prescription-strength Advil and oral hormones. I'm happy to say it worked. She stopped missing school, her grades climbed, and she was soon back to her old self. Her only regret was not coming to see me earlier. Don't let that happen to you. Remember, you deserve to feel great every day—not just three weeks a month.

One of the very best ways to make sure that happens is to make friends with your period, in all the ways we've talked about in this chapter. When you understand how your body reacts to your period every month, then you can adjust your life accordingly. If you notice that you break out before your period, don't just wait for the zits. Try ramping up your skin-care routine a week or two *before* your period comes. If you always feel exhausted for the first few days of your period, schedule in some extra sleep.

If you're worried about embarrassing leaks, skip the white pants. And if you know you're going to be irritable, try to plan a nice reward for yourself—like a girls'-night-in with your best friends and favorite chick flicks. Overall, the more proactive you can be, the better you'll feel and the happier you'll be.

CHAPTER 4

ITCHES IN YOUR BRITCHES?

Dealing with Injuries, Infections, Oozing, and Bruising

There I was on the beach in Jamaica, basking in the tropical sunshine, when my daughter, Chloë, then five, came sprinting toward me from the water like Jaws was snapping at her heels.

"MY BAGINA'S ON FIRE! MY BAGINA'S ON FIRE!" she shrieked.

OK, so at age five, she hadn't mastered her "V" sounds yet. Still, I'm sure everyone on the beach understood her perfectly. Part of me wanted to slink behind the nearest palm tree. The gynecologist in me, however, wanted to stand up and cheer. She knew the right terminology!

It turned out the salt water had irritated the delicate skin of her private parts. Luckily, all it took was a little Vaseline, begged from a nearby mom with a diaper bag, to soothe the burning. "I'm never going swimming again," Chloë declared.

Ten minutes later, she was back in the water.

Most of my patients don't burst into my office shouting, "My vagina's on fire." But a few of them probably wish they could. Not a day goes by—*not one single day*—where one of my teenage patients doesn't beg for help with itching, burning, or some funky vaginal discharge. So if you thought you were the only one squirming in agony during English class (and not just because Hemingway's a bore) or wondering who slimed your underwear, don't worry. You're not alone.

In fact, itching, pain, and discharge caused by vaginal infections are some of the most common problems affecting teens and tweens. Luckily, they're also some of easiest to treat. That may not sound terribly comforting when you're wondering whether it's better to die from itching, or die from embarrassment at the doctor's office. After all, chances are good that the doctor will actually have to *look* at your problem. Maybe it would be better to ignore it and die with dignity, right?

That's one option. But if you've read this far, I hope you've realized that seeing a gynecologist is no big deal, even for problems that seem embarrassing. Remember, for doctors like me, there's nothing at all embarrassing or awkward about all this. Like I always say, to me, looking at a vagina, even an itchy one, is like examining an ear, nose, or throat. Just another day at the office.

In this chapter I'll give you the low-down on problems down low—infections, irritations, and even piercing problems. I'll also tell you how to care for injuries to these oh-so-tender parts.

WHAT'S GOING ON DOWN THERE?

In general any irritation, swelling, or discomfort to the vagina is called vaginitis. If your symptoms are itching, burning, and discharge, chances are you have one of these three problems.

Yeast. This might sound gross, but yeast, whether it's in your sandwich bread or in your vagina, is actually a fungus. Yep. Like a mushroom. With all the TV ads for anti-yeast creams and the huge aisle of yeast-control products at drugstores, you'd think yeast was taking over the planet. But lots of other things can cause itching and irritation, too, so don't just run out for an over-the-counter remedy.

I hadn't seen my patient Kristin in a while, until she called and asked for an emergency appointment last spring. Her vagina was so irritated she could hardly walk. She'd been using over-the-counter medication for itching, but it only gave her brief relief (see the box on page 78 about why those creams do more harm than good). When she hobbled into my office, she looked so sick I thought her appendix might have burst.

When I examined her, I didn't see any common signs of infection. Her vagina was clean as a whistle. No clumps of white, cottage cheesy-type discharge. No redness. No swelling. Nada. Zip. Totally normal. But she obviously was suffering, so I did a culture and treated her for yeast anyway. It turned out she did have her first yeast infection—even though her only symptom was itching. She felt better in one or two days and started walking like herself again. Lesson: Take yeast infections seriously . . . and see a doctor if you're itchy, uncomfortable, or in pain.

DID YOU KNOW?
Young Girls Don't Get Yeast Infections

Most healthy young girls will *not* experience vaginal yeast infections. Yeast needs estrogen to really thrive, and prepubertal girls just don't have enough estrogen circulating through their bodies to provide a feast for the yeast, so it doesn't settle in.

The good news about yeast infections (if there *is* any) is that they're usually easy to treat. Often all it takes is one little pill called Diflucan. The medication gets into the bloodstream and launches a seek-and-destroy mission on yeastie beasties. Most girls start to feel better in a day or two. Just to be sure, I usually repeat the dose three to five days later, to make sure the critters are really gone and won't come back to torture you.

Another treatment is vaginal creams, which you squeeze into the vagina using an applicator that looks like a skinny tampon. These creams normally are applied for three to seven days at bedtime. I don't usually prescribe creams for teen girls for two reasons: First, the medicines have substances in them that can actually be *more* irritating to an already sensitive area; and second, who in the world wants a gloppy mess in her vagina when she's already having issues? My motto: Most of the time, the less you put in your vagina, the better.

YEAST: DR. ASHTON'S HOME REMEDY

Plain yogurt with live active cultures in it can help you avoid and even treat yeast infections. That's because some yogurts—those with *L. acidophilus*, or live active cultures—help keep yeast in your body from running amok. The "culture" in yogurt is actually a good bacteria (but what marketer would ever put "live bacteria" on a yogurt container?). The yogurt's bacteria battles it out with the yeast and the winner is your vagina. Here's my home remedy for yeast infections:

INGREDIENTS

- Plain, unsweetened yogurt (with no flavoring—and no sprinkles on top!) containing active cultures
- One tampon

Dip the tampon in the yogurt, insert, and leave in for one to two hours.

Some of my patients swear that *eating* yogurt with live active cultures helps them avoid vaginal yeast. I don't agree. There's no secret passage from your intestines to your vagina, so there's no way for the good bacteria to find its way from your digestive tract to your privates. Still, I say, do what seems to work for you!

Strep. Yep, strep. It isn't just for throats. Although I'm willing to bet you'll never, ever hear anyone say they have "strep vagina," the same bacteria that causes strep throat is the most common cause of vaginitis in younger girls. It's not as common as yeast for teens, but it can still cause itching and discharge. Typically this bacteria causes a creamy, white vaginal discharge with no odor. Meanwhile, the outer opening of the vagina and the area around the anus typically turn bright red and become very raw-looking. Especially if you've recently had strep throat, then strep could be a leading suspect in your infection. The usual treatment is penicillin or another antibiotic.

Dermatitis. Sounds like you should see a skin doctor for this one, right? Actually, dermatitis is a general term that covers any skin inflammation—including the delicate skin between your legs. Dermatitis usually doesn't cause discharge or odors. But it does cause nonstop low-level itching and occasionally bumps. Not fun. Of course, you have no way of knowing whether this itching is caused by dermatitis, a yeast infection, or something else, so go see a doctor. A huge range of things can provoke dermatitis: Salty sea water can be one—that's what sent Chloë screaming up the beach in Jamaica. But lots of other things can bring it on, too: sitting in a bubble bath too long; harsh laundry detergents; chemicals in panty liners or tampons (which is why I recommend organic tampons—see chapter 3); and activities like exercise, swimming, or sex. Even soap can provoke it. And cleansers designed to wipe out bacteria or fend off zits can come on a little too strong for your privates. I recommend a baby soap or shampoo for washing between your legs.

 DID YOU KNOW?
Feminine Itch Creams Hurt More Than Help

No!! Stop!! No matter how much itchy agony you're in, do not—I repeat, DO NOT—use over-the-counter feminine anti-itch creams available at drugstores. I am not kidding about this. These creams may provide temporary relief, but they also include many known chemical irritants that can actually make you more uncomfortable in the future. These chemicals are a veritable recipe for the itchy-scratchies. Do not fall into this trap. Try Vaseline or Aquaphor. If those don't work, see a doctor.

INFECTION DETECTION: WHAT YOUR DOC NEEDS TO KNOW

You can help make your doctor's visit short and sweet if you do a little detective work on your own. Notice the following and be prepared to tell your doctor.

DISCHARGE: WHAT COLOR IS IT AND DOES IT SMELL BAD? As I like to tell my patients, if it isn't green, itchy, or smelly, and you're a virgin, there's usually nothing wrong.

HOW MUCH DISCHARGE IS THERE AND WHAT DOES IT LOOK LIKE? I'm not suggesting you make this into your biology class science project, but be ready to describe the basics: Is there a lot or just a little? Is it thick, thin, or clumpy? Is there an odor?

DO YOU FEEL ITCHING, BURNING, OR PAIN? When? All the time? When you pee? When you exercise? Are there other triggers?

IS IT "OUTSIDE" (THAT IS, ON THE VULVA) OR "INSIDE" (THAT IS, IN THE VAGINA)? Sometimes patients tell me they have itching in their vagina, but the affected area is really the vulva. As I tell my patients, you can think of them as different states in the same country—closely situated but different topography.

ARE THERE OTHER PHYSICAL PROBLEMS AROUND THE SAME TIME? Nausea, vomiting, diarrhea?

HOW LONG DO THE SYMPTOMS LAST? Weeks? Days? Hours? If this happens often, are there any factors related to flare-ups? Like does the itching happen more in summer months (when you may be spending time in wet swimsuits)? Do you feel itchy when you're exercising and wearing certain clothes?

> **DO YOUR PRIVATES LOOK RED, SWOLLEN, OR IRRITATED?** Use a mirror to check.
>
> By now you'll have collected enough info to be able to give a very thorough description to your doctor. Boy, will he or she be impressed with your medical presentation!

WHEN TO SEE A DOCTOR

Sometimes vaginitis clears up on its own. You can always wait a few days and see if things get better. I always tell my patients: Serious problems rarely go away by themselves. So if something clears up on its own, it probably wasn't anything to worry about.

But if you're very uncomfortable, there's no need to wait: You may feel better, sooner, if you see your doctor. In any case, if you have itching, burning, unusual discharge, or other symptoms for more than one week, or if they happen several times a year, you definitely should see a doctor.

At a visit for vaginitis, you can expect the doctor to do the following:

1. **Take a medical history.** The doctor will ask the who-what-when-where of your problem, so your detective work (see the box above) will make things quicker and simpler.
2. **Do a pelvic exam.** The doctor will look at the vulva and inside the vagina.
3. **Order a lab test.** The doctor might do a bacterial culture, which sounds a lot scarier than it is. He or she very gently rubs what's basically a Q-tip on the infected area. You'll hardly feel a thing (and I'm not just saying that because I'm a doctor and that's what they teach us to say). Later a lab tests the sample to see if any bacteria grows from it in a twenty-four-hour period. (This part really *is* a science project.)
4. **Prescribe a treatment.** Sometimes a doctor can make an edu-

cated guess as to what's causing the itching or discharge and might prescribe an antibiotic even before the culture results are back. Other times your doctor may choose to wait until the test results show you have an infection, then prescribe something.

DON'T DIS DISCHARGE

Nobody likes the word "mucus." Especially in relation to her underwear. But mucus is good. Let's say this together again: *It's the job of your cervix to make mucus.*

Let me explain why this is a good thing.

At the top of your vagina, on the lower part of your uterus, is your cervix. As I explained in chapter 1, the cervix is the gatekeeper for your reproductive organs. One of its big jobs is to protect your uterus from all the bacteria that normally live in the vagina. One way it does this is by producing a lot of mucus, which acts like a quicksand pit. It traps the bacteria so they can't climb up into your uterus. The other job of your cervical mucus factory is to lubricate and moisten the vagina, which is a good thing for sex and reproduction. When your cervix stops making mucus, it means you're in menopause. So in a strange way, you should be *happy* to see some mucus once in a while.

How do you tell if your mucus is normal? Normal discharge is subtle: It doesn't make a big dramatic scene and there's not a whole lot of it. It's just kinda there sometimes and not there other times. If you're not sexually active (which means you have NEVER, EVER had sex—not even once), any discharge that's not green, smelly, or itchy is usually normal. Yellow, white, or clear discharge is almost always OK. Large amounts of oddly colored discharge are *not*.

If discharge bothers you, try charting it. Note on a calendar the days when your mucus level seems high or low. (You can add this to your period calendar—see chapter 3 for instructions.) Finding that your body's mucus factory has a specific production schedule might make you feel better. It's good to make friends with your normal discharge. Then you'll recognize when something is wrong.

BV (or Pee-Yew!). You'll recognize this one right away if you're familiar with your usual inoffensive friendly discharge. BV, for bacterial vaginosis, is usually associated with sexual activity, but not always. I mentioned it in chapter 2, but it's worth another mention here because it's so very annoying and common. If you have it, you'll know it: It produces a lot of grayish, thin, slimy discharge with a nasty, fishy odor. Blech! Your vaginal area might itch, too. BV is caused by an overgrowth of some types of bacteria found in the vagina—the most common type is called *Gardnerella*.

Your doctor can easily diagnose BV with a quick office visit or a Q-tip test. The treatment is pretty simple, too. You apply a prescription antibiotic cream to the vagina, in either a single dose or for several nights in a row, using a narrow plastic applicator. Or you can take an oral antibiotic, although most doctors prefer the vaginal route. Unfortunately, BV can be like a pesky ex-boyfriend: It keeps showing up at the worst times. Sometimes patients need to take antibiotics for one week of every month for several months until these persistent little bacteria finally take the hint.

 DR. ASHTON'S ITCHY-SCRATCHY PLAYLIST

- Never, ever use over-the-counter creams for vaginal itching. They do more harm than good.
- If it clears up on its own, you're probably OK. Serious problems rarely just go away.
- If you're a virgin and have discharge that's not green, smelly, or itchy, there's usually nothing to worry about.
- It's the job of your cervix to make mucus: When it stops, you're in menopause.

THINGS THAT GO BUMP

One day my patient Elena came in looking grim.

"I have a sexually transmitted infection," she announced.

"Really? How do you know?" I asked.

In the shower she'd felt strange bumps in her bikini region. When she looked in the mirror, she saw an alarming rash.

"Let's take a look," I said. I stepped out of the exam room while she put on a snuggly patient robe. When I came back in and examined Elena, we were both relieved to learn that all she had was a hair follicle with a major infection. The culprit: shaving. The cure: warm soaks and a topical antibiotic. Problem solved.

As Elena found out, it's pretty alarming to be minding your own business in the shower, getting yourself squeaky clean, when you suddenly notice a bump down there. But fear not. Most of the time strange bumps in your groin will be from one of three common causes.

Folliculitis

- **What it looks like:** Tiny zitlike bumps, usually red, in the pubic hair region. Small but sometimes quite painful. Often they have a little pus in the center.
- **What causes it:** As I mentioned in chapter 2, these little pimply bumps form when pubic hair follicles get inflamed or infected.
- **What to do:** Do *not* squeeze or pop them: This could spread the infection to the surrounding skin. A few times a day, press a warm washcloth to the bumps for a few minutes to help relieve the pressure and pain. Your doctor can prescribe an antibiotic lotion for them if they really bother you, but often they clear up on their own. Pay close attention when grooming pubic hair (see my advice for avoiding folliculitis in chapter 2).

Insect Bites

One patient came to see me after she found a painful red bump in her groin. I took a look. The raised bump surrounded by a circle of red skin turned out to be a tick bite. She'd contracted Lyme disease. I prescribed antibiotics for three weeks and she was fine.

Sometimes we forget that ticks, mosquitoes, and other insects can find their way to your tender parts, just like anywhere else on your body. Unfortunately, bug bites in the genital region can be very prone to infection, since there's a lot of bad bacteria nearby in the rectum and because it's the kind of dark, moist hangout bacteria like best.

> **What it looks like:** A bug bite. But it might get even redder and more swollen if it's infected.
>
> **What to do:** See a doctor. When it comes to bumps between your legs, if it's red or itchy, or if it hurts, get it checked out by a health-care professional.

Moles and Beauty Marks

Skin is skin. If your arms, legs, and face can get a mole, beauty mark, or skin tag (which is another little skin growth), so can your vulva and vagina. Of course, you may not be in the habit of *looking* down there much, so if one day while showering you feel something unusual, you might freak out. This is another reason why it's good to make friends with your personal anatomy by taking a good look at the vulva and vagina every so often with a mirror. Then you'll know if something changes or appears out of the blue.

> **What it looks like:** Slightly raised areas of skin, often darker in color than the surrounding skin. If irritated by underwear or friction caused by sports, sex, or other activities, moles or marks might start to bleed.
>
> **What to do:** If a mole or mark is bleeding or seems to be growing or changing, see a doctor. They usually are benign, but it's possible for skin cancer to appear in the genital region—although usually this happens in much older women, not teens.

Hidradenitis

Hidradenitis is an uncommon skin disorder that produces large, painful boils and leaves scars. It is not sexually transmitted or associated with sexual activity.

What it looks like: Big, painful, pus-filled lumps. Usually found in groups, often near areas with a lot of sweat glands, like the groin or under the arms.

What to do: See a skin specialist or dermatologist.

? TRUE OR FALSE?

Thongs Cause Yeast Infections

FALSE. Thongs do *not* cause yeast infections. If they did, half the women in America would be squirming in their seats. So bring on the string. But, obviously, if you already have a yeast infection or other irritation, thongs might, er, rub you the wrong way, so to speak. If so . . . try good old-fashioned cotton briefs. Nobody has to know. It's better to wear granny pants than suffer. And remember, it's a great idea to bare it all at night; letting your vagina feel the breeze while you sleep can help you avoid infections.

PIERCING[10]: READ THIS BEFORE YOU PIERCE ANYTHING (EVEN YOUR EARS!)

My patient Lauren, who's sixteen and comes from a well-off family in the 'burbs, dropped by recently for a routine visit. As soon as I started the exam, I noticed something had changed. She'd had her clitoris pierced. Some things you just can't keep secret from your gynecologist.

Now, I see a lot of things as a doctor, and many of them hurt. Injuries. Operations. Diseases. I myself have broken bones playing sports, had two babies, and (worst of all) passed two kidney stones. So I'm a person who's familiar with pain. But this looked like something even *I'd* rank high on the agony scale.

"Hmm," I said to Lauren. "That must have hurt."

"Oh, yeah," she said, wincing. "I wish I'd never done it." She'd tried to remove it but couldn't get it out.

"Want me to take it out?" I offered. She said yes, and a few seconds later I handed it to her. She tossed it in the trash can.

"That was a big mistake," she said. I asked why she did it.

"My ex-boyfriend and some friends talked me into it. I was scared, but I didn't want to be a wimp." She didn't know it would hurt so much for so long. She'd done it secretly and was embarrassed to talk to her parents about it. By the time it stopped hurting, her boyfriend was ancient history. She hated to imagine what her future boyfriends would think about it.

Lauren certainly wasn't the first patient I've seen with a genital piercing, but she was one of the youngest. Now, I'm not a person who judges my patients. I've said it before—I'm no prude, and I'm not a judge, priest, or rabbi. If adventurous piercing never caused anybody any emotional or physical harm, I'd have nothing to say here. But it's my job to keep you healthy and make sure you know about the risks. And the fact is, with genital piercing, you risk permanent damage to your anatomy that can ruin your future sex life.

THE HOLE STORY

Lauren sure wasn't the first girl to feel pressured into piercing. Actually, most teens who go in for body piercing get the idea from friends or acquaintances. (It's not like your cute old granny's going to suggest one.) A lot of teens who get pierced aren't all that good at the whole "just say no" thing: Teens who pierce their bodies tend to have higher rates of drinking, drug use, and sexual activity.

On one hand, exotic piercings seem like a daring, wild, nonconformist thing to do. On the other hand, everybody else is doing it (so maybe it's not such a nonconformist thing after all). Somewhere between one in three and one in ten American teens have some part of their body pierced, according to estimates . . . and we're not talking earlobes. In college students the percentage estimate goes as high as 50 percent.

Whatever the case, if you're thinking—even for a minute—about piercing your nipples or genitals, you absolutely must know five things.

1. **Piercing is surgery.** All surgery has risks. The risks for piercing include infection, bleeding, and damage to the area or nearby anatomy. And when I say infection, I'm not talking about irritating little bumps. I'm talking HIV, hepatitis, tetanus, nasty bacterial infections—major, life-threatening infections. These infections can and sometimes do travel to your heart, bones, kidneys, bloodstream, or joints. You could end up in the hospital or with lifelong conditions as a result. Plus, *any* infection in a genital piercing could result in trouble with your sex life, recurring genital pain, or even problems urinating for the rest of your life. You'd never suddenly decide to have surgery without mulling over the risks and benefits. And you certainly wouldn't get surgery on a dare. So treat piercing like the surgery it is—not like an impulse buy.

2. **Different body parts take different times to heal.** While your piercing heals, you might not be able to swim, and you might have oozing, discharge, and pain for a *long* time after the procedure.

HEALING TIME FOR PIERCINGS:
- Ears: one to two months
- Nostril: eight to twelve weeks
- Labia: Up to four months
- Navel: four months to one year
- Nipples: six to twelve months
- Tongue: four weeks

3. **Genitals are not ears.** Perhaps you've noticed this yourself. Different anatomical parts are prone to different reactions to piercing. Earlobes aren't a big deal: They take a while to heal, but hardly anybody loses an ear after piercing. If you have a bad reaction to a genital piercing, however, you may suffer the results for the rest of your life. The clitoris is especially vulnerable to scarring, infection, and allergic reaction. Worse still, because the blood supply to the clitoris can be damaged during piercing, the nerve and skin can partially or completely die. This could take away the pleasure of sex and actually make it painful for the rest of your life. Something to think about.

4. **Piercing parlors are like restaurants.** Some are clean and sanitary. Some you wouldn't want your dog (or even your older brother) to eat at. If you've decided to get a piercing, look for a licensed parlor with an approval certificate posted on the wall from the local or state department of health and the Association of Professional Piercers. Find out how much experience the piercer has. You do *not* want to be a guinea pig for a nipple or genital piercing. Also, many reputable places will not perform a piercing on anyone under the age of eighteen without an adult accompanying them, so realize that this is not something that you should do without your parent's knowledge. ID is required in most places. Going behind your parents' backs to a place that doesn't require ID for your age is like *asking* for an infection.

5. **Check out www.safepiercing.org.** Here you'll find information about safety and hygienic practices and standards. Read before you let anyone punch a hole in you.

INFECTED PIERCINGS

So let's say you've done your homework and really thought hard about body piercing for a long time. You're not out at the mall with friends, you're not doing it on a dare, and you've talked to your parents about it. Even if you do everything right, something still could go wrong. If you think you have an infection after piercing—if you have redness, extreme pain, green discharge, or a fever—proceed immediately to a doctor. Do not pass Go; do not collect $200. Don't waste time seeking out the guy who did the piercing or talking to your friend who got pierced. You need a doctor or nurse to look at it right away, even if it's embarrassing.

PIERCING DOS AND DON'TS

Do: Keep the piercing in place, even if it gets infected. I know, it's counterintuitive. Seems like you'd want to remove the problem, right? But, actually, taking out the stud or ring would cause the hole to close up, trapping the infection inside and under the skin, which can be even worse. Most problems can be solved without taking out the piercing.

Do: Use warm compresses for a few minutes on the infected area several times a day.

Do: Wash with mild, antibacterial soap several times a day.

Don't: Use ointments of any kind, including antibiotic ointment, around new piercings. Ointments can clog up the site and trap bacteria inside.

Don't: Use hydrogen peroxide, alcohol, or Betadine for aftercare. These can kill good skin cells as well as bacteria.

DID YOU KNOW?
Tongue Piercing Can Be Tasteless

Tongue piercings pose risks that other piercings don't. Some of these risks are dangerous, like airway obstruction, hemorrhaging, or problems with safely chewing and swallowing. Some are annoying, like the danger of chipped teeth. (My good friend and dentist, Patti, gets a lot of business because of tongue piercings.) But there are two risks that would *really* bother me: Piercings can damage taste buds, so you may lose some of your sense of taste. And potential nerve damage to the tongue causes problems with your speech. Since talking and eating are two of life's greatest pleasures, be sure you understand the risks before you let someone punch a hole in your tongue.

GENITAL TRAUMA: FIRST AID FOR FRAGILE PARTS

Speaking of piercings, did you ever see that episode of *Grey's Anatomy* where a patient's genital piercing gets stuck in his ex-wife's diaphragm while the two are in a compromising position? Meredith and her colleagues have to separate them, guided by X-ray images. That's not exactly something that happens every day (OK, ever) in my office. But if I were a writer for the show, I'd definitely have enough material for a few appalling episodes on genital trauma. Like . . . did you know that boys and men can actually fracture their penis? I've seen it in the emergency room, and it's seriously one of the worst injuries I've ever seen in my medical career. Usually this occurs during sex (with an erect penis) and is a major emergency requiring surgery.

Luckily, we ladies can't break our vulvas or fracture our vaginas. But that doesn't mean genital injuries aren't common among women. They are, but nobody talks about them. I get calls all the time from other doctors about patients who suffered an injury "down there."

"Down *where?*" I ask myself. "Their knees? Their feet? Come on, let's be *doctors* here." If other physicians feel uncomfortable with this part of the anatomy, it's easy to understand how the average teenage patient feels.

Statistics on genital injuries are scarce, and since they're not exactly the kind of thing girlfriends text each other about, you may not realize how common they are. Chances are you know somebody who's suffered a painful fall off a bike or a sports mishap that left her bruised between the legs. And while everyone takes genital injuries to boys seriously—that's why they wear athletic cups—these injuries often are dismissed, overlooked, or undertreated for girls. True, girls' genitals may be better protected than boys'. But they're just as sensitive and very vulnerable to injury. Because they get so little attention, you need to be aware of the dangers and what you can do if you hurt yourself.

EVERYTHING YOU NEVER WANTED TO KNOW ABOUT GENITAL INJURIES

What dumb movie would be complete without a scene where some poor guy takes it in the soft parts? Somehow comedy writers just won't go there with women, but the injuries are every bit as painful. Especially for girls, tweens, and teens, whose anatomy is more easily injured than that of grown women.

This is true for three reasons. First, there's much less fat tissue in the vulva of girls than in that of grown women. Like a bumper car with no padding, this area lacks the cushioning that protects the external and internal genital structures on a grown woman. So even a simple fall can cause much more damage for a girl than for an adult. This is also a region on the medical map that we doctors called "highly vascularized"—in other words, it has some major-league blood supply, so even little cuts can bleed *a lot*.

Second, the three important openings in young female genitalia are much closer together than they are in an adult. The urethra, where the urine comes out, the vagina, and the anus are all very close to one another. In adult anatomy the openings are more spread out. That means, for girls, an injury to one opening is more likely to affect the other openings. If a woman slips and falls in the bathtub, injuring her urethra (where the urine comes out), the problem may only involve that particular structure. But in a preteen it could easily involve the vagina as well.

Third, tweens and prepubescent girls don't have estrogen circulating in their genital tissue, like mature teenagers and adult women do. As it turns out, estrogen is a powerful promoter of healing in the tissues of the female genitalia. That's why we heal so quickly after childbirth, even if we've had cuts or tears to the delicate tissue down there. And it's why doctors often prescribe low-dose estrogen cream for girls with genital injuries, to help them heal faster. (Sorry—estrogen's rapid healing effects are confined to the vulva and vagina. It doesn't help you heal any faster elsewhere on your body. So don't expect to find estrogen-infused Band-Aids anytime soon.)

IT'S A GIRL THING: HOW YOUR ANATOMY IS DIFFERENT WHEN YOU'RE YOUNG

- Less fat tissue
- Important openings are closer together
- No circulating estrogen to help healing

WORST CASE SCENARIO: WHY PREVENTION BEATS TREATMENT

It was a sunny day in April. Jessica, an eleven-year-old girl, was romping on the school jungle gym during recess when she slipped and slammed down hard on the bar, right between her legs. Howling in pain, Jessica was rushed to the nurse, then a nearby emergency room.

Inexplicably, the hospital sent her home. To this day I don't know why. Maybe her doctors asked her to open her legs, and she couldn't because of the pain. Maybe the blood obscured their view. Maybe the doctors simply didn't feel comfortable treating young girls' anatomy, so they weren't thorough.

Whatever the reason, they clearly didn't give her a careful exam. Eighteen hours later, after an agonizing night, Jessica came to my hospital, still bleeding and in pain. I took her directly to the operating room. When we put her legs in the stirrups, we were horrified. The fall had ripped away all the skin in her pubic area: We could actually see the white pubic bone. And we could barely identify any normal anatomy.

Luckily, we were able to repair Jessica's soft tissue in the operating room. She spent several days in the hospital on pain medications with a catheter draining her urine. Eventually she healed very well.

Fortunately, most girls won't suffer this kind of dangerous genital accident. But it shows you how easily these things can happen—and how serious they can be.

HOUSE OF HORROR! A GUIDED TOUR

So now you're thinking, "That's all very interesting, Dr. Ashton, but this kind of injury just isn't going to happen to me." Maybe not—but let's take a quick tour of your house, shall we? I'll point out a few dangers you might not have spotted, so you can be on the lookout, while I tell you about the four most common genital injuries.

Let's start in the bathroom. I've seen some scary injuries result from a simple slip. Got a sliding glass door? Those metal tracks can act like razor blades during a fall, resulting in a laceration, or cut, to the genitals. Even a wide porcelain bathtub rim can cause a significant blunt injury—which may swell, bruise, or even bleed—if you slip and land on it in a straddle position. Hence the name for an injury resulting from a hard landing between the legs: a straddle injury. And watch out if your younger siblings still play with pirate ships, pots and pans, or superheroes in the bathtub: You know how much it hurts just to *step* on one of those? Imagine falling and landing in the wrong place.

That's why I've told my daughter since her toddler years to be extremely careful getting out of the tub. She gets it. She knows one slip could result in a bad injury to her "bagina."

Let's move on to the kitchen. You're late for soccer practice, but you need your favorite water bottle. It's on the top shelf and there's no time to get a stepladder. You hop on a kitchen chair. If you stretch just a little bit . . . you balance on one foot . . . and . . . boom! Suddenly you and the chair topple over. As the chair falls, you land on a corner of the seat, or the arm, or worse . . . one of the chair legs.

This kind of fall often leads to a soft-tissue injury. These are basically bruises that may include swelling. This is one more reason I try to stay out of the kitchen. (Just kidding.)

You see the risks . . . and so far we haven't even tried anything dangerous yet.

By now you're probably getting the point, so to speak. Most girls aren't going to slam down on the gym bars and sustain the kind of trauma my poor patient Jessica did. But anytime you're playing, jumping, running, or falling—anytime your legs aren't closed—the genital region is vulnerable to even the smallest impact. Gymnasts and softball players are especially prone to genital injury.

Water sports and water play can inflict their own brand of especially painful injury, called insufflation. This type of genital trauma happens when water and air are rapidly, forcefully pushed into the vagina at a high speed. Because the vagina is a hollow and limited space, the water or air has nowhere to go, so it kind of pops like a balloon to relieve the pressure inside. This can cause a tear almost identical to what we see in the labor and delivery room. To avoid this type of injury, keep your legs together when jumping or diving, and wear thick shorts or a wetsuit when waterskiing or at a water park.

One more word on water injuries: sprinklers. I cared for a nine-year-old who slipped on wet grass, landed on a sprinkler, and ended up with a three-inch gash on her labia. I'm going to sound really evil here, but I don't let my daughter play in the sprinkler. I've seen too many accidents to feel happy watching any girl run on wet, slippery grass and jump over a pointy metal object. I suggest you cool off under the hose instead.

Play hard, play safe. Don't get me wrong: I'm not saying you should stay inside and do needlepoint all day. I *want* you to play actively and test your physical limits. That's critical for your physical and emotional development. But I want you to avoid injuries that don't have to happen. Make your environment safe and anticipate possible accidents before it's too late.

 DR. ASHTON'S "OW-THAT-HURTS!" PLAYLIST

- Protect your privates!
- Play hard—but be aware of things that could injure you between your legs.
- When waterskiing or enjoying other water sports—even at waterslides—wear thick shorts.
- Keep your legs together when jumping or diving into water.

YOU DID WHAT?! WHERE?!

You may not have heard of these injuries, but they're very common.

- **Straddle injuries:** Caused by a hard fall or bump between the legs.
- **Lacerations:** Cuts and tears, usually bleeding.
- **Soft tissue injuries:** Bruises and swelling—may indicate more serious internal damage.
- **Insufflation:** A cut or tear in the vagina, similar to a childbirth tear, caused by overinflation of the vagina by water or air under high pressure (often caused by jumping into a pool or going down a water slide).

GENTLE GENITAL FIRST AID

So what do you do when you're actually faced with one of these injuries? First, be prepared for drama. Wailing, screaming, panic. From your mother. Parents really freak out about these things. Then remember these six things.

1. **Stay calm.** That will help your parents stay calm, too. Fortunately, since you've read this book, you'll know what to do.
2. **Be prepared for blood.** Lots of it. More blood circulates around the genital region than around, say, your hands, arms, or legs, so, like scalp wounds, they tend to bleed a lot.
3. **Stop the bleeding.** Grab a towel if there's one handy, or use your shirt if there isn't. Apply direct pressure to your crotch, about as firmly as a good handshake. If you use too little pressure, the bleeding won't stop. Too much and it could worsen the injury causing the bleeding.
4. **Don't look!** As you apply pressure, *do not look!* Don't give in to the temptation to keep checking on the wound. Don't keep applying and removing the cloth. Just keep that firm pressure on until medical personnel can take over. When the bleeding's under control, get to an emergency room. Any genital wound with a lot of bleeding should be evaluated immediately by a physician.
5. **Ice it.** If you're *not* bleeding, apply an ice pack to the injury. (A bag of frozen corn or peas wrapped in a T-shirt also works great.) This will keep down the swelling so it doesn't hurt so much later.
6. **Eyeball it.** Often an injury won't seem that bad at first, but bruising and swelling makes it more painful the next day. If so, it's a good idea to take a look. It's easiest to do this with a hand mirror, while lying on a bed with your heels together, knees flopped open, like a yoga pose. Are there any cuts, any bleeding, any bruises, or any swelling? Be ready to describe what you see to a

doctor. One good way to describe the location of bruising or cuts is to imagine the numbers of a clock around the area, with the anus in the six o'clock position and the pubic bone at the twelve o'clock position. Your doctor will also want to know where your pain is located (outside, inside, etc.). After any genital injury, pay attention to whether you can pee: If you can't, this could be a severe internal injury.

AT THE HOSPITAL

If the injury involves a lot of bleeding or seems scary in some way, head to the emergency room. When you get to the hospital, the doctor will need to have a good understanding of how the injury happened. As doctors, we have to make sure you haven't been abused, so the medical staff may ask questions that seem weird or out of line. They might even question you and your parents separately depending on how old you are. Please don't take this personally—it's our job to protect you.

After finding out how the injury took place, the physician will clean the area and perform an exam. Even just the cleaning may be enough to make you scream: Sometimes these injuries are so painful that they just can't be examined while you're conscious. In that case the doctor probably will ask to put you under deep sedation or general anesthesia. This is usually a good idea. It will spare you a lot of pain and offer you the best chance of a safe, complete exam, where the doctor can assess all your internal and external structures. That's what we did with Jessica, my patient who slipped on the jungle gym. While she rested under sedation, we could take a close look at her injuries and quickly figure out what she needed.

Most genital traumas aren't severe, nor do they require major medical attention. But it's a whole lot better to overinvestigate an injury than to dismiss it, only to see it become a serious problem later on.

1. If the injury is bleeding at all. For heavy bleeding, call 911.
2. If you can't pee within a few hours of the accident.
3. If you feel OK, but the accident seemed scary and dangerous—a fall from a twelve-foot-high jungle gym, a collision on a bike at high speed, or anything that seems like it could cause a serious injury.

TAKE TWO ADVIL AND TRY SOME FROZEN CORN

If your doctor says your injury is minor, you're lucky. You can manage the pain with ice packs (again, I recommend a bag of frozen corn wrapped in a T-shirt), which help a lot in the first twenty-four hours after an accident. Treat superficial cuts or scrapes with antibiotic ointment. And, of course, Advil and Tylenol can provide mild pain relief.

IT COULD BE WORSE: YOUR MOTHER COULD BE A GYNECOLOGIST

By now you've probably learned way more than you ever wanted to know about female genital trauma. Just be glad I'm not your mother. Last week I had to run out from the kitchen to stop my kids and their three friends, all girls, from hurtling down our steep driveway while sitting astride their Razor scooters. "Stop!" I yelled. "See that bar between your legs? See that curb you're going to run into? Get it?" I exclaimed. "Trust me, I'm a doctor. You have to protect your privates." It's not fun being Mean Momma (and it's even less fun, and way more embarrassing, for my kids!). But trust me—it's better than a trip to the emergency room.

CHAPTER 5

BEAUTY AND THE BREAST

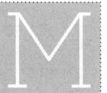y patient Carole, seventeen, called my office one morning after a sleepless night.

She told my nurse, Anna, that she'd found a huge lump in her breast before going to bed the night before. Anna made her an emergency appointment and Carole came in right away. I expected to find either an abscess (a lump of pus that develops inside infected tissue) or a benign cyst known as a fibroadenoma, which is common in teenagers.

When Carole arrived, I checked her breast while she sat upright on the exam table. Everything looked fine. I didn't see any odd dimples or redness suggesting an infection. Then, with Carole lying down, I examined both breasts. She showed me where the lump was.

I felt something, all right: The upper ridge of her chest muscle! Specifically, one of her pectoralis muscles (you know—the "pecs," which you build up when you lift weights). It turns out that in a young, strong female, these can feel . . . well, hard. Maybe even a little lumpy. Everything was OK.

Carole was hugely relieved. So was I! And I was proud of her for examining her breasts and calling me right away when she thought something wasn't normal. Learning what your breasts are supposed to feel like is one of the most important things you can do for your body in your teens: If you know how they feel when they're healthy, you'll know right away if something's *not* right.

By the time you finish this chapter, you'll understand much more about your breasts, what they should feel like, and what to do about some common problems.

BREAST BASICS

Our culture is obsessed with breasts: Why else would we have a restaurant chain called Hooters? Some of my patients can't wait to fill in. They start designing their dream wardrobe the second they get their first training bra.

But there's more to breasts than meets the eye. As you can tell right from the very first time you examine your own breasts, there's a lot going on in there. You'll feel muscles and masses and bumps and ducts and all kinds of things that can make you worry. As I said above, our job is to learn what your breasts feel like when they're normal and healthy (see the box on breast exams, page 112).

In chapter 2 we talked about the stages of breast development, from flat, to buds, to mounds (with the nipple on its own little mound), to full adult shape. Most girls' breasts have reached their full adult size and shape by around seventeen or eighteen. Here's what your breasts contain.

NIPPLES. Large, small, smooth, bumpy, dimpled/inverted, flat, pointy—it's all normal. So is a wispy hair or two near the nipple (the pointy part that contains many small openings for milk to come out during breast-feeding) or the areola—the raised, colored area around the nipple.

BREAST MOUND. Made up of muscle, fat, glands, and ducts. Large or small, the mound of flesh beneath the nipple contains some amazing equipment. The breast mound is actually the world's most efficient factory for the healthiest baby food imaginable—breast milk. Scientists still don't understand all the beneficial compounds and elements found in breast milk, but

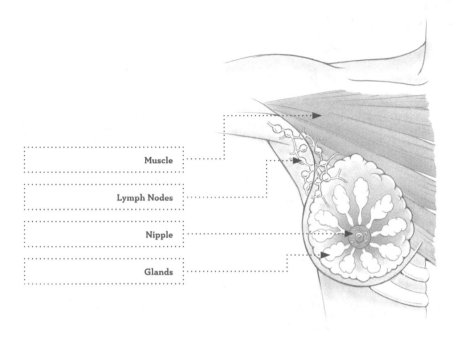

Muscle

Lymph Nodes

Nipple

Glands

they do know that breast-fed babies are in many ways healthier than those fed on formula. So even as a teenager, long before you have a baby, your breast tissue doesn't just feel like normal fat and muscle—you can feel the somewhat irregular glandular tissue, too.

When you're pregnant, your body converts most of your breast fat into glandular tissue. The milk ducts become more intricate. By the time you have your baby, your breasts are ready to produce milk.

LYMPH NODES. These glands, under your arm and your collarbone, produce lymph, a clear fluid that travels through your arteries and helps keep tissue throughout your body firm and healthy by filtering out bad cells. Lymph also travels through your breasts and drains through your lymphatic system and lymph nodes.

BREASTS 911

Since breast tissue is so different from other parts of the body—as well as so important to your body image—my patients find *a lot* to worry about. Here are a few of the worries I hear every week, along with a less common question or two:

"I've got one baseball and one golf ball!"

Your friendly neighborhood shoe retailer probably has told you that most people have one foot that's slightly larger than the other. The same is true for breasts. In fact, it's considered normal to have one breast be up to 1 1/2 inches in diameter bigger than the other. But while lopsided breasts may be normal, convenient they're not. Just try finding a bra that fits when one breast is an A cup and one is a B cup. This happened to my patient Courtney, whom I mentioned in chapter 1. When she was in her early twenties, she decided to have implant surgery to make them a matched set. She feels much less embarrassed and self-conscious now (and she spends a lot less time searching for comfortable bras!). If you're worried that your breasts are lopsided (and about 25 percent of girls do worry about that[11]), my advice is to wait until you're around eighteen. If the asymmetry still bothers you then, talk to your doctor about surgery.

"My breasts look like a circus tent!"

Red stripes? White stripes? You're probably seeing stretch marks—one or more streaks in white, gray, pink, red, or purple on the sides of your breasts, hips, or other parts of your body that are growing rapidly. You may get them again later on if you have a baby. Beware of products that promise to remove stretch marks: All the creams in the world won't work. The good news is that, with time, they'll fade in a big way. If you're very self-conscious about your stretch marks and they don't fade with time, ask your doctor about laser surgery, which can be very effective in removing some stretch marks.

"Ouch! My boobs are killing me!"

Life is so unfair. For years you look forward to developing a chest like Angelina Jolie when she was breast-feeding her twins. Now, you'd gladly go back to your pancake days, if your chest would just stop hurting. Sorry, this is a one-way trip.

Would it make you feel any better to know that breast soreness (which doctors call mastalgia) is totally common? Not much? Well, at least the pain *doesn't* mean you have breast cancer, which is something many of my patients ask me about. "Trust me," I tell them, "if pain were a major symptom of breast cancer, there'd be a lot more early detection."

Instead mastalgia often comes and goes, usually linked to your menstrual cycle. What in the world do your boobs have to do with your period? They respond to changes in your body's hormone levels, especially to the two main female hormones, estrogen and progesterone. So you might notice more breast tenderness in the two weeks before your period, when your hormones are at high tide. And you'll probably notice pain equally in both breasts. (By the way, the fact that both breasts hurt is a clue that nothing's seriously wrong. It's pretty unlikely that you'd have a major problem with both breasts at the same time.)

But just because pain is common doesn't mean you have to live with it. A few things you can try:

- In the two weeks before your period comes, cut back on caffeine. Caffeine causes blood vessels to dilate, which causes swelling and can make the pain worse.
- Take Motrin or Advil.
- Try 1000 milligrams a day of supplementary magnesium. Don't take more—too much is dangerous.
- Eat less fat in your diet. Temporarily reducing dietary fat to less than 15 percent of your total intake can be helpful in the long term.
- If your breasts are a B cup or larger, try sleeping with a fitted tank top for extra support.
- A low-dose birth-control pill sometimes can also lessen breast pain linked to your period, by keeping your hormone levels steady.

"My breasts tackled a soccer ball (or a lacrosse stick . . . or a kitchen door . . .) and lost."

With girls participating in more active sports than ever before, it's no sur-prise to hear that breast injuries are on the rise. An elbow to the breast in soccer or a stick to the chest in lacrosse usually just leaves a bruise, easily treated with ice packs and Advil. But occasionally an injury to the breast can turn into a breast abscess. This painful and dangerous infection hap-pens when bacteria enter one of the tiny openings in the nipple and attach themselves to deep breast tissue. To bacteria, anywhere warm, dark, and wet—like the inside of your breast tissue—is basically a luxury resort. Once they check in, they're hard to kick out.

When bacteria enter your breast, your body tries to protect itself by forming an abscess—a pocket of pus around the bacteria, in between the fat and muscle cells in the breast. If you develop an abscess, you might find a tender lump or hard area in your breast or see streaks of red on your chest that look like sunburn. You'll probably feel a lot of pain and you may run a fever or feel body aches. If you have these symptoms, especially if you've had a breast injury recently, see a doctor right away. A sonogram or ultrasound can show whether you have one. To treat it, a breast surgeon might drain the abscess with a needle or make a small opening in the skin over the breast. Meanwhile, you'll take antibiotics to prevent the infection from getting worse.

"Is this a nipple . . . or a belly button?"

My patient Sasha had inverted nipples: The pointy tip that usually turns outward turned inward instead, like an "innie" belly button. This is per-fectly normal and won't cause health problems: It's not even a big problem for breast-feeding. Still, Sasha didn't love the look, and she asked me about cosmetic surgery. Inverted nipples generally don't respond very well to surgical repair, but I referred her to a plastic surgeon. Sasha is now weighing the risks and benefits of an operation. She says she feels better just knowing what her options are.

"What's this stuff coming from my nipple?"

Your breasts aren't supposed to leak liquid until you're breast-feeding. So if you have any discharge at any other time, see a doctor right away. Usually it's not anything nasty, but it could be an infection, which should be treated before it gets worse.

Your doctor will ask these questions: Does the discharge emerge only when you press firmly on your nipple or breast? Or does it come out all by itself, with no pressure? Does it involve one or both breasts? What color is it?

If the discharge is milky white, it might actually be . . . milk. Certain medications or a hormonal imbalance involving the thyroid can cause milk leaks like this. To figure out what's causing it, your doctor probably will run blood tests for hormones called prolactin and TSH, and might order an MRI so he or she can study your pituitary gland. If an underactive thyroid is causing the problem, medications can treat it.

If the discharge is bloody or brown, you might have an infection in the duct system. If the infection is severe enough to cause bloody nipple discharge, you'll probably also have other obvious symptoms, like pain, redness, and swelling. In this case, your doctor probably will prescribe an antibiotic and order a sonogram. In older women dark discharge can also suggest growths in the duct system—but this is very rare in teens.

Happy Birthday: Enjoy Your Implants!

How's this for a Sweet Sixteen present? New boobs. Teen breast implants are becoming more and more common—even though many reputable surgeons won't enlarge (or "augment") breasts of girls younger than eighteen. In 2007 almost 8,000 girls eighteen and under had breast enlargements, and about 4,200 had breast reductions, according to the American Society for Aesthetic Plastic Surgery. This is a huge increase over the past decade.

But at around $4,000 a pop, wouldn't you really rather put a down payment on a car?

Fortunately, research says that about 75 percent of girls are satisfied with the size of their breasts.

Still, magazines, movies, TV, and the Internet (and, oh, I don't know, maybe the Hooters chain?) all put a lot of pressure on us to measure up. Some 40 percent of girls say media images of celebrities influence how they feel about themselves. And for some of my patients, breasts really do cause acute embarrassment or inconvenience, like my patient Courtney's unmatched set. So I understand why some girls want a couple extra birthday balloons in their bras.

But I also know the risks involved with breast enlargement. As I always tell my patients, there is no such thing as minor surgery. *Anytime* someone decides to go under the knife, regardless of how minor the procedure, there are risks involved. In the case of breast augmentation surgery, these risks include:

General Anesthesia. To receive implants, you'll be "put to sleep" with either intravenous (IV) or inhaled medications. Since you basically stop breathing, you'll be put on a breathing machine (ventilator) with a breathing tube placed down the trachea. That's at least a little traumatic for your body. Only about 1 in 500,000 people die per year due to general anesthesia—but that's one too many if it happens to be you. Especially since you didn't have to have this surgery: It's not like your appendix had to come out or it might rupture and kill you. We're talking about bigger boobs here. Nobody ever died from small breasts.

Infection. I met Julie, age nineteen, the day after she had breast implant surgery. Her doctors had called me into the hospital to consult on her case after she developed septic shock—a condition that happens when infections spread in the body or blood and sends the patient into shock. Julie had a very high fever, a racing heart, and dangerously low blood pressure. She was admitted to the ICU in critical condition. A surgeon removed the implants, but the bacteria spread to her skin and the muscle covering her abdomen. She needed several more surgeries. At one point the doctors gave her only a 50-50 chance of survival. She pulled through—but now she has permanent scars, from her breasts to her groin. All that for bigger breasts.

Re-operation. As much as 5 percent of the time the skin, muscle, or fat around an implant becomes scarred and hardened. Known as a "capsule formation," this looks gross and feels awful. The only treatment is to remove the old implant and replace it with a new one. This means undergoing all the risks of surgery again.

"Come on, Dr. Ashton," you're saying. "Tell us how you *really* feel about breast implants for teens."

OK, so I'm not exactly shy about my opinions. But in case you haven't guessed yet, I don't think it's a good idea to get breast implants in your teens. Yes, technically your breasts are usually physically mature by the late teens. But your body image is not: That continues to mature and develop until your early twenties. Like it or not, feeling insecure about your body during your high-pressure teens is the rule, not the exception, and getting comfortable with your body—its beauties and its imperfections—is part of growing up. In my opinion, this is *not* the time to start changing your body like you change your clothes or your hairstyle. If you do, you might miss out on an important growing experience—one that doesn't involve a cup size. I'm talking about the growth of your spirit, your person, your self-image, and your self-esteem. These things can't be bought and they can't be surgically implanted.

? TRUE OR FALSE?

Breast implants have an expiration date.

SORT OF TRUE. Many implants will need to be replaced or redone in ten to fifteen years, which requires another operation.

Breast implants or reduction surgery may affect your ability to breast-feed your baby later in life.

TRUE. Breast-feeding brings big benefits to babies, so talk to your surgeon about implications for breast-feeding.

Small Wonders: Breast Reduction Surgery

Alexa, eighteen, and her mother came to see me the summer before Alexa's senior year. As with all my new patients, I asked why she'd come in. Was it "just the right time" to see a gynecologist? Was she having problems with her period? Was she thinking about becoming sexually active? No, no, and no.

I must admit I was a bit perplexed, until Alexa burst out with the big news. "I'm here because my plastic surgeon needs a gynecologist to do a real breast exam on me before my surgery next week." Aha!

She told me she was having breast reduction surgery and she couldn't wait. With her beautiful mother sitting right next to her (who'd had breast reduction surgery about a decade before), Alexa told me how her DD-cup breasts interfered with her life on a daily basis. She felt very self-conscious wearing anything but baggy sweatshirts. When she played tennis with her high school team, she felt like she had two extra players bouncing around on the court with her. Plus, the weight of her breasts really hurt her back.

Breast reduction surgery is one type of elective surgery that I feel **can** be a good idea, even as early as eighteen, because large breasts can cause pain and other physical problems. In addition to unwanted attention and back pain, teens with large breasts can develop skin problems in the area under the breasts, including yeast infections (yep, yeast can grow there, too). And when breasts hang and sag, they can rub and chafe the skin, causing pain and discomfort.

By the age of eighteen, your breasts have pretty much reached their adult size and shape, so in my opinion, it's a reasonable age to consider corrective reduction surgery. Yes, it does present almost the same risks as breast augmentation surgery, so talk to your doctors and parents before sprinting off to the operating room. Remember, there's no such thing as minor surgery. Still, unlike breast augmentation, breast reduction *can* provide real relief for real physical problems, as Alexa's mother reminded me.

"I wish I'd done mine much earlier," she told me. "I don't want Alexa to suffer like I did."

 QUIZ: IS THIS NORMAL?

Which of these is normal for teenage breasts?

   A. One breast to be larger than the other
   B. Red streaks or dimples after an injury
   C. A few hairs around the nipple
   D. A hard, round lump like a pea or marble below the skin
   E. Occasional breast pain or soreness
   F. Leaking liquid from your nipples
   G. To have a lump that's getting bigger
   H. To see changes in the skin on your breast

ANSWER: A, C, and E are normal. B, D, F, G, and H are not. See a doctor if you experience any of these.

HOW ARE BREASTS LIKE A TV REMOTE?

Let me tell you a personal breast story (no, not "personal best"—just the opposite, actually). At age twenty-nine, I was in medical school and had my first baby, Alex. I knew breast-feeding would help my baby in all kinds of ways and reduce my risk of breast cancer later in life. So I definitely planned on breast-feeding. In fact, I was actually a little insulted when the breast-feeding teacher walked into my hospital room after Alex was born and asked if I had any questions. I mean, how tough could it be? I had breasts, Alex had a mouth, milk would come out, and there you have it. "I'm a med student, for cryin' out loud," I thought to myself. "I think I can figure it out."

"No thanks," I told the breast-feeding teacher. "I've got it totally under control."

Back home with Alex, I quickly regretted my words. It turns out that breasts are a lot like complicated TV remotes: Just because you *have* them doesn't mean you know how to *use* them.

I didn't have a clue how to get Alex to eat, and he didn't either. Before I knew it, my little guy had lost too much weight because he wasn't getting enough milk. I was terribly worried about him, not to mention that I felt like a failure. In fact, in my hormonal state, I had a major freak-out. Of course, now I know that lots of moms and babies struggle to get it right. (And with my second baby, I didn't send the breast-feeding teacher away! I begged for more tips! I read books, I took lessons, I talked to friends. The second time was a breeze.)

The moral of this story: Having a body part does not guarantee you know how to use it. Just like having a complicated TV remote is no guarantee you'll know how to switch from satellite TV to DVR to DVD. Simply having breasts doesn't mean you'll necessarily know what's normal and what isn't: You have to practice and explore and get to know your own breasts. You have to learn how to do your own monthly breast exam and know what's a lump and what's just normal, glandular, duct-filled tissue. Learning to care for your breasts is one more reason to see a gynecologist in your early teens. Gynecologists do dozens and dozens of breast exams every week, and they really know what's normal.

BREAST EXAMS 101

Get in the habit of giving yourself a breast exam on a regular basis. I recommend doing it a week or two after you get your period, since breasts can be more tender or bloated during your period. You don't have to become obsessive about it or do it like clockwork, but you should know what your breasts feel like when they're healthy.

Examining Your Breasts

1. Examine your breasts when you're lying down and when you're standing up. Your breast tissue falls differently depending on your position.
2. Check yourself in the mirror when you're getting in or out of the shower. Lift your arms straight over your head. Look for an unusual dimple or indentation in the skin of your breast. Then put your hands on your hips and look for the same things. (Don't worry if your breasts are different sizes; that's normal—see above.)
3. While lying down, bend one arm over your head, and use the opposite hand to gently feel around the breast on that side of your body. Feel around your entire breast, around your nipple, into your armpit, and up around your collarbone. You're looking for anything that feels hard and round, like a pea or marble, or any nipple discharge. Also notice anything that feels new or different from last time. Repeat the same exam on the other side.
4. Do the same thing standing up: Many women do this in the shower.

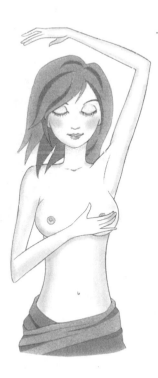

5. If you find lumps or bumps, call a doctor. But *don't* worry too much. Breast cancer in teens is almost unheard of. Teens do sometimes develop cysts (ducts or glands in the breast tissue that get stretched out with fluid), which sometimes become quite large. While definitely stress-producing, they are *not* related to cancer. Sometimes a minor surgery is required to remove them.

6. Don't be embarrassed to ask your doctor about anything strange, bumpy, or lumpy that you feel. Breast tissue isn't like any other tissue on your body, and it can feel irregular and even lumpy at first. Show your doctor what you're concerned about, and get to know your body.

HOW OFTEN SHOULD YOU EXAMINE YOUR BREASTS?

There's no hard and fast rule about how often you should examine your breasts. In fact, there's some controversy in the medical world about whether or not women and teens should routinely examine their own breasts at all. On one hand, it's important to know your body and what it feels like. And many women do find lumps during self-exams that turn out to be breast cancer.

On the other hand, the cold hard numbers show that self-exams do *not* reduce death from breast cancer and lead to many unnecessary tests and biopsies that turn out to be nothing.

The American Cancer Society's official position is that checking your own breasts should be "an option." OK. So what does that mean? Most doctors, including me, still encourage it. I want my patients to know as much about their bodies as possible—and examining your breasts is an important step in that direction. "You don't have to do it all the time," I tell my patients. "But you should do it often enough so you know how to do an exam, and you know what your healthy breasts feel like." Some doctors recommend adult women check their breasts once a month after their period. Other doctors feel an annual breast examine conducted by a physician is adequate. Check with your doctor.

❓ TRUE OR FALSE?
Breast Test

Tight bras can cause breast cancer.

FALSE. Some people believe that tight bras can restrict lymphatic flow around the breasts and contribute to cancer. But no scientific evidence supports the idea that going braless reduces cancer. Meanwhile, there are lots of good reasons to wear a well-fitting bra. For instance, girls with larger breasts need support to avoid pain. In fact, some find sleeping with a light bra reduces breast pain.

Rubbing breasts increases their size.

FALSE! To whichever boy thought of this one, I say, "Nice try."

Breast-feeding will make your breasts saggy and ugly.

FALSE. They might be a little less perky after breast-feeding, since they got bigger then shrank again. But these changes are often not dramatic. And they're not much worse than the changes that come with normal aging. Plus, the benefits of breast-feeding are huge, for both your child and you.

> *Breast-feeding your children helps reduce the risk of breast cancer.*
>
> **TRUE!** Remember this a decade or two from now, when the time comes to have kids!

 DID YOU KNOW?

Breast cancer in adolescents is incredibly rare. But occasionally teens with leukemia or lymphoma develop breast tumors if the cancer spreads. Examine your breasts regularly, and if you feel something that worries you, tell someone!

YOUR PERSONAL PINK RIBBON: WHAT YOU CAN DO TO FIGHT BREAST CANCER

You've seen them everywhere: on breakfast cereals, granola bar wrappers, Triscuit boxes, and T-shirts, as earrings, pins, necklaces, you name it. It's the pink ribbon, raising awareness for breast cancer, which is the most common type of cancer affecting women and the second leading cause of death of women in the United States, after heart disease. More people today survive than in the past, but still one in eight women will contract breast cancer during her lifetime. Seventy-five percent of girls ages eight to eighteen know someone with breast cancer. You may be one of those girls, and that may translate to a lot of worry—even though the average age of actually getting breast cancer is sixty.

Consider this section your own personal pink ribbon, raising your awareness of the risks and what you can do to avoid breast cancer.

Nothing will guarantee that you won't get breast cancer . . . just like wearing a seat belt won't guarantee that you won't get hurt in a car accident. Some things, like your family's history of breast cancer, simply can't be controlled. But there *are* things you can do right now, and throughout the rest of your life, to make it less likely that you'll get breast cancer. Living a healthy lifestyle and having regular health and wellness visits with doctors are two easy things you can do to try to lower the risk of getting breast cancer later in life. Here are some more:

1. **Learn as much as you can about your body.** This includes learning how to do breast self-exams. Although the national recommendations are to start checking yourself at age twenty, I recommend my patients start performing regular self-breast exams in their teens. This isn't to find cancer—there are virtually zero cases of breast cancer in girls under twenty. But teens can and sometimes do get benign breast cysts—exams help find them. And most important, exams help you get to know your body—and knowledge is power!

2. **Exercise regularly.** Studies suggest that six hours a week of exercise may reduce your risk of getting breast cancer by 23 percent.[12] Exercise that you do now, as a teen and young woman, may protect you decades from now. One study[13] shows that exercising moderately for as little as four hours a week earlier in life, long before breast cancer appears, could dramatically lower the risk of dying from cancer. If you were a runner in high school in your twenties but then stopped, you'd still enjoy better survival odds years later. So put on those jogging shoes now to improve your odds later.

3. **Don't drink alcohol.**[14] At your age you shouldn't be drinking anyway. To the long list of reasons not to drink, add the fact that the more you drink, the higher your risk of getting breast cancer. Don't drink before you're twenty-one, and even then, drink only occasionally and moderately—never more than two drinks a night.

115

4. **Maintain a healthy weight.** Being obese causes all kinds of health problems. It also increases your risk of getting breast cancer, possibly because fat tissue affects hormone production, and high exposure to estrogen is related to breast cancer.

5. **Take vitamin D$_3$.** Older teens should take an additional 1000 units of vitamin D$_3$ if their physician says it's OK. Vitamin D$_3$ has been linked to lower risk for breast cancer, and women who don't get enough vitamin D$_3$ have been shown to be at increased risk of breast cancer and many other diseases, too.

RISKS YOU CAN'T CONTROL

One in eight women will get breast cancer sometime during her life. But some things can make your risk even higher. In addition to some of the factors I mentioned above, like drinking alcohol and having a vitamin D$_3$ deficiency, other things can increase your risk, too.

- If your mother, grandmother, or aunts had breast cancer, you might carry a specific genetic mutation, making it more likely you'll get breast cancer.
- White women have higher breast cancer rates than African-American women.
- Women who got their period earlier are at higher risk (because exposure to estrogen is linked to breast cancer, and the earlier you hit puberty, the longer your body has been exposed to estrogen).

"Oh, great," you're thinking. "My grandmother had breast cancer and I got my period really young." Don't worry—having risk factors doesn't mean you're guaranteed to get breast cancer. But knowing you do have more risk factors, you should work even harder to exercise, maintain a healthy weight, and make other healthy choices within your control.

TO TEST OR NOT TO TEST? WHAT TO DO IF YOUR MOTHER HAD BREAST CANCER

My patient Claire, fifteen, was terribly worried about her mom, Kathy, who'd been diagnosed with breast cancer a few months earlier. Kathy had found a pea-sized lump when doing a self-exam and had seen her doctor right away. Fortunately, they'd caught it very early, which dramatically boosted her chance of survival. Still, Claire felt sick with worry for her mom, her family, and even a little for herself.

"Will I get it, too, Dr. Ashton?" she asked.

Claire's chances definitely were higher than average. I told her about all the preventive things she could do to reduce her odds of getting breast cancer (see above).

I also advised her *against* one thing until she's older: genetic testing. Today tests can tell whether you have a specific gene mutation that dramatically increases your risk of developing breast cancer. But I don't think getting these tests is a good idea until you hit your mid-twenties.

"If the tests show you *don't* have the mutation, you'd feel a little better," I told Claire. "But it's still not a guarantee you won't get it. And if you *do* have the mutation, you'll feel stressed and anxious, and there won't be anything to do about it." Since Claire, at fifteen, was already doing everything she could to prevent cancer, by exercising most days, eating healthfully, doing regular breast exams, and, of course, avoiding alcohol, knowing she had the mutation wouldn't help her.

On the other hand, I did recommend that she get tested in her mid-twenties. If she tests positive for the mutation at that point, she'll be able to take some actions. She could start having ultrasound or MRI screenings of her breasts, or think about preventive surgery (some women at very high risk of breast cancer have their breasts removed and replaced with implants). If she wants to have children, she might think about having them earlier rather than waiting—since, if she gets breast cancer later, her treatment might make it more difficult to conceive. Claire will have options and choices at twenty-five that she doesn't have now.

Although there are no formal guidelines for this, Claire's doctors probably will start formally screening her, with ultrasounds or other tests, when Claire is ten years younger than her mother was when she got cancer. (Claire's mom was forty-five, so she'll probably start having ultrasounds, mammograms, or MRIs at age thirty-five.) If your mother had breast cancer, be sure to talk to your doctor about your concerns, and do all you can to reduce your risks. But I recommend waiting on the genetic tests until you're in your mid-twenties.

? TRUE OR FALSE?

Using deodorant increases the risk of breast cancer.

FALSE. This persistent rumor hasn't been confirmed by any formal or rigorous study. Plus, it just doesn't make sense. If deodorant caused cancer, why would it cause only breast cancer and not other cancers? And if you *stop* using deodorant, you may have a whole new set of problems—social ones.

Taking the birth-control pill causes breast cancer.

FALSE. For more than fifty years, since the birth control pill was invented, doctors have studied women who take it to see if they're at higher risk for breast cancer. Although some studies say yes and some say no, most doctors now believe that adult women (not teens) who take birth control pills have a slightly higher rate of *detection* of breast cancer. That doesn't mean they get it more often, but that they *find* it more often—probably because these women see their doctors more often because they're on the pill. Their risk of detecting breast cancer falls back to normal after they stop taking it.

Bottom line: Conclusive studies don't show increased risk of breast cancer. If you need to be on the pill, most physicians and patients alike feel that the benefits outweigh the risks.

BREAST IN PEACE

Understanding and taking care of your breasts is such an important topic that I could write a whole book on breasts. But I don't have to! There's already a great one out there. I recommend you read *Taking Care of Your "Girls": A Breast Health Guide for Girls, Teens, and In-Betweens* by Marisa Weiss, M.D., and Isabel Friedman. Why worry when you can learn the facts? Knowledge is power!

CHAPTER 6

NO BONES ABOUT IT

Deposit Now or Never

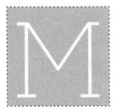any of my patients are serious athletes. Soccer players, runners, tennis players—girls who do three sports a year and get recruited by Division I colleges. These are girls who understand the power of their bodies. They know the importance of hard work and practice. They know that being athletic makes them cool and confident in a million ways.

What these girls *don't* always know (until we talk about it) is that all that running, jumping, and playing might actually save their lives—by helping them avoid osteoporosis when they're in their seventies and eighties.

"Oh, come on, Dr. Ashton," you're saying. "Why are you telling me about an old ladies' disease?"

How about this? Because osteoporosis can kill you. Not directly, like cancer or heart disease. But the bone weakness and increase in fractures that result from osteoporosis contribute to a huge number of deaths of older women. In fact, older women who fall and break a hip due to osteoporosis have a 25 percent chance of dying the year after the injury—that's one in four! And for older women osteoporosis leads to more days spent in the hospital than for many other diseases. A whopping one in three women (and one in five men) will be affected by osteoporosis in her lifetime.[15]

OK, enough bad news. The good news is that *right now*, while you're a teenager and before you hit twenty-five, is *the only chance you'll ever have* to beef up your bones for life. Right now your body is still able to deposit calcium and build very strong bones. But that's only true until your mid-twenties. After age twenty-five all you can do is try to avoid losing bone—you can't build it up no matter how much milk you drink.

Fortunately, you don't have to be a super-athlete to reap this bone bonanza (bone-anza?). Even regular walking or moderate jogging a few times a week can help. The important thing is that you start paying attention to your bone health *right now*. You can't make up for it later. In this chapter we'll bone up on how to build healthy bones for life.

 DID YOU KNOW?

Many doctors now consider osteoporosis a pediatric disease! Not because there's an epidemic of kids hobbling around with canes but because what we do for (or against) our bones when we're young determines how healthy or sick our bones will be sixty years or so down the road.

 DR. ASHTON'S GOOD BONES PLAYLIST

- Between now and the time you turn twenty-five is the *only chance you'll ever have* to deposit more calcium and make your bones stronger.
- What you do for your bones now may keep you alive and thriving when you're in your sixties and beyond.
- Exercise, exercise, exercise! (Oh, and did I mention exercise?)

YOUR BONE BANK

Imagine that the rules of banking changed overnight. Suddenly you're only allowed to deposit money in your savings account until you reach age twenty-five. After that you can *never make a deposit again*. All the money you spend in the next sixty or seventy years will be withdrawn from that account, from money you saved before you turned twenty-five. In that case I'm guessing you'd do everything you could to build up that bank account right now.

That's exactly the way your bones work. Calcium is the cash you deposit to make them strong. But once you're about twenty-five, you can't deposit any more. The growth plates that cause bones to grow close up. So consider me the Suze Orman of bone savings: Follow my advice, make lots of deposits now, and you'll be calcium-rich and fabulous for the rest of your life.

BONE BUILDING—FACTORS YOU CONTROL:
- Healthy eating (Eat dairy, sardines, almonds.)
- Dietary supplements (Take calcium and vitamin D—see below.)
- Exercise (Do weight-bearing exercises, like running or weight lifting, most days.)
- Lifestyle choices (Don't smoke or consume a lot of caffeine.)

BONE BUILDING—FACTORS YOU DON'T CONTROL:
- Family history (If your mom has osteoporosis, you're more likely to have it, too.)
- Ethnic background (Asians and Caucasians are at higher risk; African-Americans are at lower risk.)

Obviously, you can't change your family history or ethnicity. But you *can* do a lot in other areas. Here's how the bone bank works and how you can save up more.

Calcium is the foundation for bone formation. It's the building block for your bones. The more you have, the stronger your bones are. As you go through your teenage growth spurt, you'll need extra calcium to support that growth and those bones. From age nine to eighteen, you need 1300 milligrams of calcium a day.[16] After eighteen you need only about 1000 milligrams, and after you turn fifty you'll need to up it to 1200. Why so much now? Growth spurts require more materials—including much more calcium.

GOT MILK? A LOTTA MILK?

My patients often tell me they don't need to take a calcium supplement because they drink a glass of milk every day.

"Oh yeah?" I say. "Do you drink more than a liter a day?" That's how much you'd need to drink to come close to the 1300 milligrams you need. And even then you'd be short some.

Most of my patients really don't want to drink that much milk after all. Especially if they get sick from drinking milk because they're lactose intolerant (this is especially common in Asian Americans, American Indians, and African Americans). Fortunately, there are lots of ways to get calcium. Salmon, firm tofu, spinach, kale, almonds, and soybeans are all great sources of the white stuff.

Still, with the high levels of calcium you need as a teen, it's tough to eat enough of it. You'd need to eat truckloads of green veggies or vats of fish to get enough in your diet. So I tell my patients to take calcium supplements. I recommend 1200 milligrams a day, taken in two doses of 600 milligrams each, morning and night. (You have to take it in two smaller doses rather than one big one, because our bodies can only absorb so much calcium at one time.)

MY SECRET SARDINE SOLUTION

Here's my favorite source of calcium: sardines. Yep. Just two little fish have 92 milligrams of calcium. Mix with a little mayo and some onions, spread on whole wheat toast, and you can practically feel your bones getting stronger. (OK, you probably can feel your breath getting stronger, too, but it's nothing a breath mint can't fix.)

 QUIZ

Which Foods Have the Most Calcium?[17]

- 1 cup of milk
- 1 cup of plain yogurt
- 1 slice of plain cheese pizza
- ½ cup spinach
- 1 ounce almonds
- 1 cup orange juice with added calcium

ANSWER: All these foods are good sources of calcium, but yogurt is tops: It has 450 milligrams of calcium. The milk and orange juice both have 300 milligrams. The spinach has 146 milligrams. The pizza has 111 milligrams and the almonds have 71 milligrams.

D Is for Density

Vitamin D is as important as—if not *more* important than—calcium for your bones and overall health. That's because vitamin D helps you absorb the calcium you eat (say, from all those sardines). But wait, that's not all! It may also help prevent certain cancers. And heart disease. And depression. And skin disorders. Impressive, eh?

Some experts think that almost half of all Americans may be deficient in vitamin D. Most teens should take an extra 800 to 1000 units a day. Too much vitamin D can be harmful, so check with your pediatrician to see which additional dose is right for you.

Smoking Is Bad for Your Back

Smoking reduces blood flow to the spine, which can lead to future problems with discs and chronic lower back pain.

Shoes Can Hurt Your Feet

Approximately 25,000 people sprain their ankles every day. Often it's because they're wearing the wrong size shoe! Try new shoes on at the end of the day, when your feet are at their largest!

Weight Loss Reduces Arthritis

Losing a little weight can be good for your knees. Twenty percent of very overweight people in their forties will develop knee arthritis! Each pound of weight lost relieves four pounds of pressure from the knees! One more advantage of being the biggest loser.

Caffeine Weakens Bones

Excessive caffeinated and carbonated beverages "steal" calcium from your bones.

SAY YES TO STRESS

Sometimes stress is a good thing. Like bone stress—asking your bones to work harder and do more. That means walking, running, lifting weights, dancing, karate, or any field sport—basically anything that puts extra weight and pressure on your bones. This *doesn't* include swimming or other water sports. Water provides resistance, which can give you a great cardio work-out, but the whole floating thing reduces stress on your bones.

Why is stress so good? It tells your bones they have a lot of work to do, so they need to get stronger. When you stress them, they start laying down more matrix, or bone tissue. If your bones were an English muffin and calcium were the butter, the bone matrix would be the nooks and crannies inside the muffin. The more you have, the more butter (or, in this case, calcium) they can soak up and store.

How much exercise is enough? Thirty to sixty minutes a day, most days, is the best thing you can do for your bones. That could be longer sessions of moderate exercise like brisk walking, or shorter sessions of more intense activities like jogging or playing basketball.[18]

But be careful not to fall into the "more is always better" trap. There *is* such a thing as too much exercise. If you're working out excessively—say, every single day for more than two hours—your bones won't get stronger. In fact, they'll get weaker. Excessive exercise combined with too few calories tells your body that there's a famine in the land, and that this is not the time to store up calcium.

Did you ever see the Pixar flick *Wall-E*? The humans who spend their whole life lounging poolside on the spaceship can't walk around on their own. It's not just because they're lazy. Living without the stress of gravity on their bones keeps them from developing the bone mass and strength that we earthlings need.

BANK ON IT: ESTROGEN AND BONES

There's one more key player in the bone-banking system: estrogen. You already know that estrogen is your personal super-hormone, affecting practically everything that happens to your body as a young woman. So this probably won't come as a big news flash, but estrogen influences bone health, too. The mechanisms are complicated, but here's the quick and dirty version.

Estrogen affects your bones in several different ways. First, it helps calcium get into your bones. If calcium is the money you deposit, estrogen is the suitcase that takes it to the bank. The more estrogen that circulates in your system, the more calcium you deposit.

Likewise, the *less* estrogen in your system, the *less* calcium your body absorbs. That's a big problem for girls who exercise too much (more than sixteen hours a week) or have eating disorders. When body fat drops too low, your body figures that food must be scarce and that this would be a very bad time to get pregnant. You stop getting your period, your ovaries don't make enough estrogen, and you don't have the suitcases you need to get the calcium into the bank. No estrogen, no calcium deposits, no bone strength. No matter how many sardines you eat.

Another thing estrogen does is send a message to your bones to slow down their growth. It's as if your calcium suitcase also carried a note to your bank managers telling them it's closing time. A year or two after you get your period, your bone growth plates "close off" and you reach your ultimate height. The more estrogen in your system, the faster the growth plates close.

Estrogen also plays one more role. It keeps you from *losing* bone mass. Through a very complicated mechanism, estrogen keeps the bone-building cells from dying, which stops the constantly occurring breakdown of bone. In that way it's like a security guard keeping all those deposits safe.

This is why old ladies have bone problems. When women go through menopause, around age fifty-one, their ovaries stop producing estrogen. So they no longer have those security guards keeping the calcium deposits inside and preventing bone loss. (Men are a whole different story when it comes to bones, since they don't have as much estrogen.)

Fortunately, since you now know the basics of bone banking, you'll be able to save up for that day when your estrogen drops.

BUILDING BACK BONES

I already knew a little bit about Allegra when she first came to see me, because she'd been referred by another doctor. Allegra, a talented artist, had been struggling with an eating disorder and her periods had stopped. By the time I saw her, she had succeeded in a long, difficult recovery and now weighed about 101 pounds—up nearly 20 pounds from her life-threatening low point. Allegra had made good progress. But she still couldn't bear looking at the scale when my nurse checked her weight.

Although Allegra definitely was doing better, her ovaries hadn't gotten the news.

As soon as she told me her periods hadn't restarted, I began to worry about her bones. If she wasn't getting her periods, she didn't have enough estrogen in her system—and she wasn't building bone density.

To see how her bones were doing, I ordered a bone density scan, which is really just a special kind of X-ray. The scan showed she did, indeed, have osteopenia—a weakness of bones that comes right before osteoporosis.

This is *not* something you want to see in a teenager. This was the only time in Allegra's life when she could be building up her bone bank account. But, instead, her disease was robbing her of what savings she had. We needed to find a way to make sure her bones didn't end up bankrupt later in life.

One option would be to put her on a low-dose pill, which might replace the estrogen that her ovaries weren't making. Until recently this was the most common treatment. But now many doctors, including me, worry that by giving such patients an artificial "period pill," we can't tell when their normal periods really start again. So in Allegra's case, I opted against the pill. Instead Allegra, her mother, and I decided she should take calcium and vitamin D supplements while she slowly increased her body weight. I also suggested she try light weight lifting to stimulate bone density without burning too many calories. She's working on it. We'll repeat the bone scan in two years and see if her bones look healthier. We all have our fingers crossed.

? TRUE OR FALSE?
Boning Up

If you break bones as a teen, you'll get osteoporosis as an old lady.

FALSE. Although fractures as an adult can increase your risk of osteoporosis later in life, breaking them as a teen doesn't. So if you have to break a bone, do it now!

Taking one 1200-milligram calcium supplement is the same as taking two 600-milligram supplements at different times during the day.

FALSE. Your body can only absorb so much calcium at a time, so you need to break it up during the day.

A bone scan hurts.

FALSE. It's just like an X-ray.

BONE BASICS

Your teen years are the only time in your life when you can build up bone density and help avoid osteoporosis. Here's what you should do:

- Exercise thirty or more minutes most days, doing weight-bearing exercises like running, soccer, karate, field hockey, or weight lifting.
- Supplement with vitamin D. After clearing it with your doctor, take an extra 800 to 1000 units a day.
- Take calcium. I recommend 1200 milligrams of calcium every day. (Note: Don't take it all at once—instead take 600 milligrams in the morning and 600 milligrams at night.)
- Maintain a healthy weight. Don't drop below a Body Mass Index of 19, or 5 to 10 percent of your ideal BMI (see chapter 11).
- Don't smoke. It's bad for your bone density—and your heart, lungs, cervix, and skin. And your breath.
- Don't drink alcohol excessively. Don't drink at all until you reach the legal age. Too much alcohol is bad for your bones, as well as your liver and brain.

These diseases and conditions put you at higher risk for osteoporosis later:

Irritable bowel disease
Celiac disease (which prevents people from digesting the gluten
   in certain grains)
Crohn's disease (an ongoing inflammation of the digestive tract)
Diabetes
Overactive thyroid
Kidney failure
Taking certain medications (steroids and antiseizure medications,
   Depo-Provera birth control, and the blood thinner Heparin)
A Body Mass Index of less than 19 (see chapter 11)
If your periods have ever stopped for more than twelve months
Smoking
Low levels of physical activity
Low vitamin D levels
Low calcium intake

OH, *SNAP*: OTHER BONE RISKS

Anorexia is just one disease that can put you at risk for bone loss—right at the time you most need to be building up bones. Chronic medical conditions or diseases that affect the way you digest things can also hurt your bones. (see the box above for a partial list).

If you have a chronic medical condition, ask your doctor about whether it affects your bones. If your mother has osteoporosis, you should also be more careful about good bone health.

If your doctor is concerned about your bones, he or she probably will send you for a bone density scan like Allegra had. It's a painless kind of X-ray of your hips, spine, and sometimes wrists.

Of course you can't change the fact if you have a chronic disease or a family history of osteoporosis. But this is the one *time in your life* when you can give your bones an extra boost.

So don't break the bank: Deposit now.

CHAPTER 7

HORMONES GONE WILD

Polycystic Ovarian Syndrome (PCOS),
the Most Common Disorder You've Never Heard Of

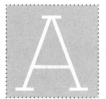shley first came to see me when she was sixteen. Her periods had been wildly irregular since they started at age thirteen, and she just couldn't take it anymore. Like most girls her age, she found it tough enough to balance school, friends, and sports. But her period seemed to have a mind of its own, coming when she least expected it—anywhere from three weeks to eight weeks apart. She never knew if it would come during an exam, a volleyball game, or a swim meet. As if her life weren't stressful enough already!

On top of all this, she had other worries. For one, there was her weight. Even though she played two sports, she couldn't get down to a healthy weight for her body. Then there was her out-of-control acne. Plus, she had extra hair on her body, especially her face. Her mom and sister, who also had excess hair, showed her how to pluck it so other people wouldn't notice—but it was one more irritation she didn't need.

Ashley wasn't exactly thrilled when her pediatrician sent her to see a gynecologist about her irregular periods. In fact, she cancelled our appointment twice before she finally came to the office. But after she and her mom had been there about fifteen minutes, she was already glad she'd come.

"OK. I think I know what's going on," I said. "If I'm right, we can help your periods, your acne, your facial hair, and your weight, too."

Ashley had no idea that all those issues might be caused by the same thing—polycystic ovarian syndrome (PCOS). Experts call this the most common but least understood hormonal disease affecting women. A whopping 10 to 26 percent of teens have PCOS.[19] Imagine ten girls in your English class. Chances are, one of them has PCOS.

In PCOS the ovaries basically work overtime, producing too much of too many hormones—particularly testosterone and something called luteinizing hormone.

I ran some blood tests and called Ashley a few days later. As the phone rang, I studied her digital photo on my Mac (I like to see my patients when I talk to them). I smiled, knowing there was a good chance that next year's photo would look a little different—clearer skin, a little less weight, a whole lot less stress. When she picked up, I told her the good news.

"Guess what? You have PCOS."

Why did I call it good news? Because when it's detected and treated, PCOS is no sweat. But undetected it can lead to a lifetime of potentially serious health problems, such as diabetes.

WHEN HORMONES RULE YOUR WORLD

Not only is polycystic ovarian syndrome an ugly, off-putting name . . . it's not even accurate! It doesn't *just* affect the ovaries—it also involves the pancreas and a bunch of other organs. And there may be no cysts at all (which are basically little liquid-filled sacks that form inside an organ). Plus, its daunting acronym, PCOS, sounds like it must be a dread disease . . . but it's not a disease at all. It's a syndrome—a collection of symptoms—which is a fancy way of saying "This is just the way your body is."

PCOS isn't something temporary that goes away, like a sinus infection. You don't catch it and then get over it, like a cold, or take a pill to get rid of it, like strep throat. And there's no single test that definitively proves whether you have it or not.

Instead PCOS is a hormonal condition you'll have for your entire reproductive life. Just as you have brown hair or blue eyes, so, too, do you have PCOS.

If you catch on and start treating PCOS early, chances are it will never be dangerous or have serious health consequences. If you don't catch it early, you might develop diabetes later or have problems getting pregnant.

WHAT DRIVES HORMONES WILD?

No one knows exactly what causes PCOS. It seems to run in families, and it might be related to obesity, since fat tissue produces hormones and can exacerbate hormonal imbalances. Whatever the cause, the main feature of PCOS is overactive ovaries and an overproduction of insulin and andro-gens (male sex hormones), particularly testosterone. (It was extra testos-terone that caused Ashley's acne and excessive body hair.) All these hormones "talk" to each other in very complicated ways, so when one is out of balance, it's a lot easier for the others to get out of balance, too. Ironically, teens with PCOS sometimes face an increased risk of preg-nancy, since their irregular cycles make it even harder to predict when they're ovulating.

HORMONE HULLABALOO?
OR TYPICAL TEEN TRAUMA?

With all these hormones running amok, you'd figure it'd be easy to diag-nose PCOS in teens. But, actually, it's easy to miss because its symptoms are so common. Irregular cycles? So what? Most teens have those at some point. Excess weight? Who doesn't struggle with a few pounds? Ditto for zits. And in this day of "less-is-more" body hair, practically *any* amount of hair can seem like too much. So girls, parents, and even their doctors often miss the warning signs of PCOS.

My patient Jane, for instance, had fairly normal periods, but she came to me as a last resort after her dermatologist had reached her zits' (oops, I mean wits') end. Sitting across from Jane at my desk, I could see that she had more than her normal share of pimples for a sixteen-year-old. When I examined her, I saw the acne extended down her back and chest. She was so embarrassed about her skin that she refused to go to the beach or a public pool.

I ran some blood tests to check her hormone levels, and sure enough, some were elevated. That, plus her slightly irregular periods, helped me to diagnose Jane with PCOS. When I brought Jane back to my office to discuss the results and what PCOS means, she was actually overjoyed that we'd figured out the reason for her bad skin. After three months on the pill, her skin was nearly flawless! *This* is why I love my job.

DR. ASHTON'S PCOS PLAYLIST

- PCOS will not affect your life as long as you're informed and manage it well.
- PCOS is not temporary; you either have it or you don't, and it doesn't go away.

SYMPTOMS OF PCOS

Having one or two of these signs doesn't mean you have PCOS. But since it's so easy to overlook, it's a good idea to mention your concerns about any of these to your doctor and ask if you should be tested for PCOS.

IRREGULAR PERIODS. This can mean never getting your first period, stopping your period for at least three months after it has become regular, having fewer than nine periods a year, or having prolonged heavy periods. Or several of the above!

These irregularities happen because the ovaries aren't releasing an egg regularly. As I mentioned in chapter 2, such anovulation, and irregular periods, can be pretty common when you first start menstruating. But if your cycles aren't predictable within four or five years after your period starts, talk to a doctor.

HEAVY BLEEDING. Anovulation can lead to periods being heavier than normal, which can lead to anemia (lack of iron in the blood).

MALE-PATTERN BODY HAIR. This might include facial hair, or hair between the breasts, from the belly button to the pubic area, or on the upper third of the thighs.

ACNE. We're not talking about a few zits now and then, but persistent, extensive acne, often including the back and chest.

OBESITY. A Body Mass Index (BMI) of 30 (or greater than than the 95th percentile for your age). To calculate your BMI, see chapter 11.

THE SNOWBALL EFFECT: WEIGHT AND PCOS

Talk about a vicious cycle. The metabolic uproar caused by PCOS can make it difficult to lose weight, even when people eat healthfully and exercise. Then the excess body weight makes PCOS worse, since peripheral body fat, also known as adipose tissue, makes estrogen, which can throw the hormone balance even more out of whack. These higher estrogen levels can eventually lead to abnormalities in the lining of the uterus—not healthy.

Plus, excess weight in women with PCOS can lead to glucose intolerance, in which the body can't process some sugars effectively. Many women with PCOS work with a nutritionist to make sure they're eating the most healthful foods for their body.

DO YOU HAVE PCOS?

If your doctor thinks you might have PCOS, here's the workup you'll go through:

CLINICAL HISTORY. Your doctor will want the story of your life. OK, not your whole life but about six months of your "menstrual history"—how often your periods come, how long they last, how heavy the bleeding is. (It's helpful to keep a period diary—see chapter 3 for instructions.) He or she will also ask about other related symptoms, such as acne and excess body hair.

BLOOD TESTS. Your doctor will test levels of two hormones made in the pituitary gland—FSH and LH, which affect the function of the ovaries, as well as testosterone levels. He or she will also test for a hormone called prolactin, which affects periods, and a thyroid hormone, called TSH (this last test is just to rule out a thyroid problem, which could cause similar symptoms). Sometimes other hormones are also tested to exclude other sources of problems. If testosterone levels are high or the ratios of other hormones aren't right, you probably have PCOS. (But . . . just to make things interesting . . . sometimes your blood tests will be normal even if you **do** have PCOS!)

BODY MASS INDEX. The doctor will take your weight and height (and maybe your waist and hip measurements) and calculate your Body Mass Index (BMI). Many, but certainly not all, teens with PCOS have a BMI of 30 or more. See chapter 11 to calculate your BMI.

PHYSICAL EXAM. Your doctor will look for unusual hair patterns—hair on your face, between your breasts, down your inner thighs, or up your lower abdomen—as well as acne and other signs of elevated testosterone. Good news—you don't usually need an internal exam for a PCOS diagnosis.

SONOGRAM. Some physicians take a sonogram (the same kind of image used to take pictures of babies in the womb) to see what your ovaries look like.

WHAT'S INSIDE YOUR OVARIES?

I did all of the above with Ashley except the sonogram. Since sonograms appear perfectly normal as much as 30 percent of the time even when patients do have PCOS, I usually don't order them.

Still, sonograms of patients with PCOS sometimes can be interesting. If Ashley's ovaries were like those of many PCOS patients, they'd be three to five times larger than average. They might also have a ring of tiny follicles around the outer rim, looking like a string of pearls.

For some patients with PCOS, a sonogram might also show one or more small ovarian cysts (hence the name polycystic ovarian syndrome). While parents and patients both get nervous when a cyst is diagnosed, cysts usually aren't dangerous. After all, when you think about it, ovaries *exist* to make cysts. The monthly process of ovulating (releasing an egg) is actually nothing more than the regular formation and subsequent rupture of a small cyst.

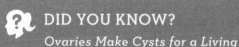

DID YOU KNOW?
Ovaries Make Cysts for a Living

A cyst is a tiny sac with fluid inside. Normal ovaries form a cyst containing an egg every month. When the cyst ruptures (tears open), the egg is released. But ovarian cysts that don't contain eggs and grow too large can occasionally cause health problems.

. . .

Usually cysts are so not a problem. Even when they show up in a sonogram, most gynecologists ignore them until they're at least 2.5 centimeters in diameter (roughly the size of your thumb joint, from the end of your nail to your knuckle). Moderate-size cysts are about twice as big, from 5 to 7 centimeters. Large cysts are 7 centimeters or bigger. Sounds huge, but even larger ovarian cysts can disappear on their own, as the fluid inside gets reabsorbed. In some cases cysts cause pain, but often they don't.

Most of the time doctors will just "follow" a cyst, taking sonograms every month or two, to see if it gets bigger or shrinks on its own. When it doesn't shrink or if it's causing pain, it may have to be removed surgically.

DON'T DO THE TWIST: OVARIAN TORSION

Sometimes when a cyst gets large, the ovary flips over and twists around its blood supply. This very painful emergency, called ovarian torsion, requires surgery right away. Often the pain, which makes it impossible to sit still or get comfortable, comes with nausea or vomiting. If you know you have a cyst and you suddenly have a lot of abdominal pain, discomfort, or vomiting, call your doctor right away.

If you do need surgery for ovarian torsion, a gynecologic surgeon will untwist the ovary, possibly remove the cyst, and leave the ovary in place, even if it appears to be "dead," with no blood supply. In the past, ovaries that appeared to have died were routinely taken out at the time of initial surgery. Today we know that ovaries can often come back to life after being untwisted, even if it takes a month or six weeks. I prefer to leave the ovary in place and follow up with several sonograms and physicals for four to six weeks after surgery. If the ovary doesn't recover, we do a second surgery to remove the dead organ. Luckily, you only need one ovary to live a perfectly normal, healthy reproductive life. But why take chances? It's nice to have a spare.

UNTREATED PCOS IS DANGEROUS

If you're diagnosed with PCOS, consider yourself incredibly lucky. If it's not caught and treated, you could have a number of serious problems later, including:

DIABETES. People with PCOS are five times more likely to develop type-2 diabetes.

HEART DISEASE. Elevated cholesterol levels can lead to cardiovascular problems.

INFERTILITY. Undiagnosed PCOS can make it much more difficult to get pregnant. When diagnosed and properly treated, becoming pregnant is usually not a problem.

CANCER. Untreated, PCOS boosts your risk of abnormalities in the endometrium (the lining of the uterus). Most of the time the lining of the uterus needs to be exposed to both estrogen and progesterone to stay healthy. As I mentioned in chapter 1, estrogen's sort of like the building blocks of the endometrium and progesterone is the cement, so you usually need both. With PCOS the endometrium gets too many bricks and not enough cement (progesterone), so there's a buildup of endometrial cells, which can lead to a precancerous condition called endometrial hyperplasia. Luckily, this is very uncommon in teens, but it can happen in women in their twenties, thirties, and older.

BALANCING ACT: HARMONIZING YOUR HORMONES

When I told Ashley she had PCOS, she was happy and relieved. Finally an answer for her period problems, body hair, and acne. When she and her mother came in to talk about treatment options, I reminded them that PCOS affected Ashley's whole body and went far deeper than her skin and hair. It's something she'll always have to manage to avoid the negatives of untreated PCOS, including fertility problems, diabetes, and abnormal cells in the uterine lining.

First, I recommended that Ashley start seeing a nutritionist specializing in PCOS. Losing weight was hard for Ashley, as it is for all patients with PCOS, but if she could take off as little as 5 percent of her body weight, studies suggest that her hormones would start to correct themselves. Ashley's nutritionist recommended minimizing certain carbs, since women with PCOS often can't process glucose effectively. So Ashley said adios to Pop-Tarts and white bread and hola to more fruits and veggies.

Meanwhile I prescribed low-dose oral hormones—the pill—which is the second most common treatment for PCOS after weight loss. Oral hormones work for PCOS for the same reason they work for avoiding pregnancy: They shut off activity in the ovaries and, instead, provide estrogen and progesterone in the correct balance.

Over the next year Ashley's acne and excess body hair were noticeably lessened. Her periods also became more regular, shorter, and lighter. With the help of her nutritionist, she took off ten pounds. She felt great. Even better, I knew the weight loss would help her body handle glucose better, reducing the risk of diabetes and high cholesterol. The lining of the uterus would also be protected from abnormal growth.

Two years later, Ashley's doing much better. But she knows that she'll have to continue to manage her PCOS for the rest of her life—it won't just go away. If she decides to have children, she'll have to stop the oral contraceptives but may get on a different type of medicine. Also, if her weight loss allows her hormone levels to normalize, she may not even need the hormone pills (as long as her periods are regular and her skin isn't a problem!).

ADDITIONAL TREATMENTS

Weight loss and the pill went a long way to helping Ashley's symptoms, so we stopped there. But those measures weren't enough for another patient, Kim, who had a more severe form of PCOS. By the age of fifteen she was already very obese and had high cholesterol. Although she and her nutritionist had worked out a healthy eating plan, she still couldn't lose weight. So I prescribed a medication called Metformin, which is often taken by diabetics. It changes the way the body handles glucose and insulin by lowering high levels of insulin and testosterone and regulating ovulation and periods in some people. (If you take Metformin and are sexually active, you also need to take the pill, since Metformin may lead to ovulation—meaning you could get pregnant, like any other girl with a regular cycle.)

Kim's doing better now, but she's still more than one hundred pounds over her ideal body weight. She's now considering Lap-Band surgery to help treat her weight, high cholesterol, and sleep problems.

STAYING IN BALANCE

It's been two years since I diagnosed Ashley, and her picture on my screen really does look different today. Clear skin. Healthier weight. But it's during her office visits when I see the real difference. She's here at least once a year for her annual cholesterol check and screening for diabetes (I usually recommend my patients with PCOS get these tests every twelve to twenty-four months). Her growing sense of confidence and control shines through whenever we talk. She's doing a great job of exercising and eating well, so her cholesterol and insulin levels are staying under control. Along the way, she's helped her mother and sister realize that they, too, have PCOS—and her entire family (including her dad and brother!) are eating better and exercising more.

All that, plus clearer skin? What's not to like?

STRAIGHT
TALK ON SEX

CHAPTER 8

THE WAIT-TILL-EIGHTEEN CLUB

Why Membership Has Its Privileges

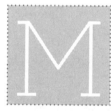y patient Sarah, a petite, wisecracking cross-country runner, came to the office three weeks before she turned eighteen. I'd seen her regularly for three years, ever since she'd come to see me about painful periods.

"Hey, Sarah, what's up?" I said, walking into the office. "Had sex yet?"

"Nope, not yet," she said cheerfully.

"Sweet!" I exclaimed, and gave her a high five. "Well done!"

Sarah was one of the last virgins in her group of smart, vivacious friends, and she was very close to joining the "Wait-Till-Eighteen" club—the 40 percent of all teens in the United States who wait until age eighteen to have sex.[20] Her decision to take a pass on casual hookups had meant she didn't date much earlier in high school. Sometimes that left her feeling lonely and out of it as a freshman and sophomore. But by junior year she was dating Tyler, a cute guy on the cross-country team.

I was thrilled she'd stood up to the social pressure for so long. But now, she told me a few minutes into our visit, the big night was on its way. She and Tyler had been dating for more than six months and she felt ready.

"It's great you've waited until now," I said. "But, look, your birthday's right around the corner. Can you please wait till then? Please? Really? Please?"

I was half teasing, half serious. After all, what difference could a few weeks make? But I wanted her to be able to congratulate herself on crossing the finish line. Why quit a marathon in mile twenty-five?

"OK, OK, I'll try," she said with a rueful grin.

And she did. Even though Tyler surprised her with a romantic dinner a few days before her birthday, she postponed their private celebration for another week. I was delighted to see the Wait-Till-Eighteen Club gain one more member. And Sarah was happy to join.

"It was a really nice feeling after the fact," she told me later, "to think, 'I feel good about this. I didn't rush into it, and I was really ready.'"

WHY WAIT TILL EIGHTEEN?

If no girl ever had an unwanted pregnancy, caught herpes or genital warts, or ended up with emotional bruises that undermined her happiness or academic success, then I wouldn't care *when* my patients had sex. As I'd told Sarah on her very first visit, I'm not your mother. I'm not here to judge you. And I'm not a prude.

But I *am* a realist. My job is to protect your health—and that's much easier if you stay a virgin until at least eighteen.

Why eighteen? No study proves you'll have a happy, healthy life if you wait. There's no American Medical Association recommended age for sex. I can't tell you there's a "safe" or "normal" age to become sexually active, and it's not my job to tell you what to think from a moral, spiritual, emotional, social, or religious standpoint. Not my job *at all*.

It *is* my job to tell you what I think from a medical and scientific standpoint. As a doctor, I know that the longer you wait, the more you lower your lifetime risk of unwanted pregnancy and sexually transmitted diseases. I know that you're more likely to be in a stable relationship with someone you really love, not a fleeting one-month crush—and that your increasing emotional maturity will help keep down the number of lifetime partners you have, further reducing your risks. Medically, I want to see you wait as long as possible. Nineteen is better than eighteen. And twenty is even better than nineteen. And so on.

So why do I say eighteen should be the earliest you should consider having sex? Because my patients tell me that eighteen sounds reasonable—and achievable. It's a nice specific goal. It's the legal age for voting, smoking, and serving in the military. And it's not *that* much longer than the national median age of first intercourse (17.4 for girls, 16.9 for boys).[21] When I explain that delaying sex can have lifelong effects on a girl's physical, emotional, and psychological health, it sounds even more reasonable.

Don't get me wrong—I know it's a challenge to wait. Nationally only 40 percent of girls get to eighteen without having sex, and that number is even lower in urban areas. In my own practice in a suburb of New York City, just 25 percent of eighteen year-old patients are still virgins. But some girls, like Sarah, succeed. And in fact, more and more girls *and* guys are waiting. Read on for more details.

What sets them apart? My brilliant advice! (Just kidding.) The truth is, girls are smart. Given the right facts, they usually make smart choices. Knowing all the medical science behind sex and having lots of support from a doctor like me, from good friends, and from your family can make it a lot easier to join the Wait-Till-Eighteen Club—and to enjoy the member benefits for the rest of your life.

WHY JOIN THE WAIT-TILL-EIGHTEEN CLUB?

MEDICALLY

- You are more likely to contract sexually transmitted infections than mature women.
- In the early teen years, your cervical cells are still developing and sex at an earlier age can interfere with normal cell development (I'll tell you more about this in the next chapter).

SOCIALLY

- If you wait longer, you're more likely to be in a longer-term relationship and have fewer regrets.
- Half of all teens who have had sex wish they'd waited until they were older, according to a study by the Kaiser Family Foundation and *Seventeen* magazine, and 25 percent of teens who have had sex would change the person they were with the first time.[22]
- Having sex early goes hand-in-hand with other high-risk activity, like smoking, drinking, or drug use. Doing one of these puts you at risk for trying the others. The stakes are too high to take a chance.

EVERYBODY'S NOT DOING IT

If you join the Wait-Till-Eighteen Club, you'll have lots of company. Fewer and fewer teens are having sex in high school: A little less than half of all high school students have had sex today.

Why the drop? For one, our culture is talking about sex more openly. Whatever you may think about Paris Hilton, *Girls Gone Wild*, and the media attention paid to so-called rainbow parties where teens swap oral sex—all that attention has at least sparked conversations. It's also led to aggressive campaigns to educate teens about sex. The thinking: If you're going to hear, see, and talk about sex, you'd better have all the facts. Since 1997 MTV has aired hundreds of millions of dollars worth of ads about safe sex and more than a million callers have phoned its safe-sex info hotline.[23] Other media campaigns targeting teens have also made a mark.

One thing that *hasn't* been shown to work: abstinence-only education. Studies have shown that preaching abstinence without teaching safe-sex practices *does not* reduce teen sex. You need all the facts—about abstinence, contraception, and safe sex—to make good choices.

In my own practice I've found several other important things that can help, too: Knowing how to talk to your doctor, your parents, your friends, and your boyfriend about sex can all make a big difference.

 DR. ASHTON'S TALK-TO-YOUR-DOCTOR PLAYLIST FOR NEW PATIENTS

I mentioned some of these back in chapter 1, but a good playlist is one you play again . . . and again . . . and again. Your doctor is the perfect person to answer all your questions and give you a little advice before the big deed is done. These tips will help you get what you need.

DON'T FEEL EMBARRASSED. If you only take away one thing from this book, I want it to be this: Please don't ever feel embarrassed or ashamed of your body. When you meet your gynecologist, go ahead—ask her anything. She wants to help you, but she can't unless she knows what's on your mind.

YOUR INFORMATION IS CONFIDENTIAL. If you tell me something confidentially, then, legally, I can't share it with your parents—unless I feel your safety or someone else's safety is at risk (in which case I need to tell your parents and possibly the appropriate authorities). There's one other exception to the confidentiality rule: If you have chlamydia or gonorrhea, the testing lab will automatically report it to the state health department.

BE HONEST. I trust you. But I don't read minds. I assume you're being honest with me about whether you're sexually active or not. If you tell me you're a virgin, I'm *not* going to give you the same exam or treatment you'd need if you were sexually active. You have to be honest with me or I can't help keep you healthy. So speak up. Tell me what you're doing. I promise I won't be shocked, disgusted, or disappointed. It's all in a day's work for me.

I don't need to do Pap smears or pelvic exams until you're sexually active. As long as you're a virgin, I probably won't need you to put your feet in the stirrups. Most of my patients find this another good reason to wait.

DEALING WITH FRIENDS

A funny thing I've noticed: Although I talk to thousands of patients every year (many of those just before or just after they lose their virginity), none of them, not *one* teenage patient, has ever said to me, "Oh, Dr. Ashton, I love my boyfriend so much, and I really want to sleep with him because it will bring us closer." Or even "Dr. Ashton, I had sex, and it *rocked*. It was *so great!*" Not once.

Most of my patients just don't see sex as a demonstration of love, affection, or intimacy. It's something they do because "the time seemed right" and because there are all kinds of social messages out there telling them it's the thing to do. Friends, music, TV, movies—all suggest that high school is the natural, logical time to lose your virginity. But a lot of those messages are pure myth. If you know the facts, you'll know how to respond to your friends when they bring them up.

Myth 1: You have to have sex to fulfill a relationship.

Truth: You don't need to have sex. There are plenty of other things you and your boyfriend can do.
I say this all the time—even when my patients' parents are in the room. Sometimes the parents just about fall out of their chairs. But the fact is, 80

percent of my patients have had oral sex by age sixteen, and most of them have engaged in some variety of sex play. Of course, oral sex and sex play won't protect you from sexually transmitted infections. (Let me repeat that: Anything you can get from vaginal intercourse you can get from oral sex. *Anything.* Warts, herpes, chlamydia, gonorrhea, hepatitis, HIV. All of it. In your throat.) Still, you won't get pregnant—and that's a big plus. And you can and should use condoms even during oral sex to reduce the STI risk (I know it sounds weird, but you really don't want to get an STI through oral sex—see chapter 8 for details).

This point—that having intercourse isn't the only way to get cozy—is a great one to use on boyfriends or friends who might be pressuring you. It shows you're not a prude (if that's something you're worried about) and it also shows you know what you're doing. Plus, it's totally in line with how most teens feel about sex. Most of my patients also don't see sex as the ultimate expression of love, or even a chance for a great orgasm (by the time they get to intercourse, most of my patients have already had plenty of experience with physical pleasure, through oral sex and other sex play). When it comes to vaginal intercourse, I tell my patients, "You don't need to check that box right now. You can do it anytime."

ALPHABET SOUP: VD, STD, OR STI

When I was a kid sexually transmitted diseases were all referred to as "VD"—venereal disease—since "venereal" means "coming from sexual intercourse." Today they're usually called sexually transmitted diseases (STDs) or sexually transmitted infections (STIs). Personally, I say "STI," because it's more accurate—a disease can come from any number of causes, but an infection is caused specifically by a virus or bacteria spread from person to person.

Myth 2: You have to have intercourse to have sexual pleasure.

Truth: You don't need to be sexually intimate with anyone to have an orgasm.

Let me fill you in on a mother's secret: Most moms of little boys (and maybe even bigger boys) downright *expect* that they'll have a hand down their pants at some time every day!

There seems to be a different standard for girls, however. I can't tell you how many times I've seen mothers reprimand their little girls for "playing with themselves." I can't tell you why this is true—that's a subject for a class on society and gender—but (surprise) I can give you my opinion: This is ridiculous. It's totally normal for girls, like boys, to explore their bodies in search of that "good feeling" that comes from touching a certain place in a certain way. This is true for a toddler, it's true for a teenager, and it's true for an adult woman. Studies have shown that 80 percent of teenage boys and 60 percent of teenage girls have masturbated by the age of eighteen. It's common, normal, and one of the few things that truly has no risks at all. Touching yourself doesn't cause psychological problems, doesn't make you a pervert, and doesn't make you go blind. There shouldn't be any areas of your body that you're afraid to touch, and you shouldn't feel there's anything wrong with you for enjoying that sensation.

In fact, something very positive can result from learning how to provide yourself with this form of physical pleasure. Whether you call it self-stimulation, masturbation, or auto-arousal, the concept is the same: YOU DO NOT NEED TO BE SEXUALLY INTIMATE WITH ANOTHER PERSON IN ORDER TO GET THIS FEELING. You can achieve these feelings all by yourself. While there certainly are meaningful social consequences that result from having a close physical relationship with someone when you are emotionally and physically ready, you should know that you don't have to seek out another person purely as a means of providing this physical feeling.

Also, by exploring your own body and how it responds to different types of touching, you may be more aware of your own sexual likes and dislikes in the future, when there *is* another person involved. And if you're wondering about orgasms (what they're like, how to tell if/when you have one, etc.), don't stress. Orgasms are different for each person but pretty easy to recognize. If you've had a really great physical feeling that starts small and gets bigger and bigger, you've probably had one. And if you haven't, keep exploring your body—you will!

JUST DOING IT: MAJOR REASONS WHY TEENS SAID YES TO SEX[24]

Curiosity (85%)

Partner wanted to (84%)

It was the right time (82%)

Was ready (80%)

Met the right person (76%)

Been with the right partner for a long time (74%)

Hoped it would make the relationship closer (69%)

Friends had already done it (62%)

Wanted to get it over with (58%)

Planning to marry the partner (53%)

Was using drugs or alcohol (18%)

Myth 3: More is better.

Truth: Keep your lifetime number LOW.

We live in a supersize society. We want bigger houses, more food, and bigger cars—no wonder our economy got into big trouble in 2008. People (that is, adults) just kept wanting more, more, more . . . until they outspent their budgets. Why was anyone surprised? At school you hear the more-more-more message constantly. The more friends you have, the better! The more activities you're in, the better! The more colleges you apply to, the better! But that's not necessarily true. Imagine if you participated in so many activities or filled out so many college applications that you didn't have time to sleep. If you've ever felt overcommitted and stressed out, then you know what I'm talking about—more isn't always better.

Unfortunately, some people want you to think that more is better when it comes to sex. That's just not true. Medically speaking, sex with more people isn't better. It's *a lot* worse. I illustrate this for my patients by showing them the "sex pyramid," which explains how, by sleeping with *one guy even once*, you may be, in effect, sleeping with dozens or even hundreds of people. (Check out the drawing on page 190.) You're exposing yourself to anything his partners have, and anything their partners had, and so on and so on. . . . That's pretty scary in a world where more than half of all people carry the HPV virus and 20 percent of Americans have genital herpes.

While *more is better* is medically false, it's also not going to make you any more popular—not in the long run. When I talk to my patients, I point out that having sex to become more popular just doesn't work. "How are you going to feel," I ask my patients, "when you have sex with a boy, and then find out he had sex with everyone else in the class? Or brags about sleeping with you on Facebook? Or texts everybody you know?" This isn't hypothetical: It happens all the time. This kind of embarrassment is the opposite of the social props teens are looking for. Most girls already know this: 84 percent of teens say that keeping the respect of their friends is an important benefit that comes from postponing sex.

BENEFITS OF KEEPING YOUR "LIFETIME NUMBER" IN THE SINGLE DIGITS

MEDICALLY

- More partners increase your lifetime risk of sexually transmitted infections. More partners and more sex increase your risk of pregnancy.

SOCIALLY

- If you sleep with one boyfriend in high school, you'll probably end up sleeping with the next . . . and all the other ones after that.
- Someday you'll meet the man of your dreams. He may feel better and so will you if you *both* have a lower lifetime number.

Myth 4: Once you've lost your virginity, you might as well sleep with all your future boyfriends.

Truth: You can become a "retroactive virgin."

Just because you have sex with one guy doesn't mean you need to have sex with every other guy you like. One patient of mine really regretted losing her virginity, so we swore a pact. She vowed not to have sex again until eighteen, and I promised to declare her a "retroactive virgin" if she made it. She did.

TALKING TO YOUR BOYFRIEND: PRACTICE MAKES PERFECT

One of the best tips I give my patients who want to delay sexual activity—but aren't sure how to resist temptation—is to be prepared. Anticipate the obstacles that may pop up in your path and make a firm plan to deal with them. Preparation is key.

Your plan might be as simple as figuring out how to say no when asked out on a date ("That's so nice of you, but I just don't have any time right now") to the trickier logistics of cooling things down when you and your boyfriend are making out. Think about what you'll say and practice saying it.

What should you say and how should you say it? I believe honesty is the best policy. Firmly and honestly tell him you're not planning to have sex until later in life, for lots of good reasons. But while I want you to be honest, I also live in the real world, and I know that sometimes it's easier to have some extra reasons, excuses, or even white lies up your sleeve. Some patients find it's helpful to offer a concrete reason: One of my patients told her steady boyfriend that her parents would buy her a car for graduation if she was still a virgin when she got her diploma. Her little white lie wasn't actually true—but it helped her to have something specific to say. After he got over the fact that he was less important to her than a car, he respected her wishes.

Thinking about situations in advance will help you handle them in a swift, confident, decisive way if they come up. If you have responses or excuses ready in your mind, you can avoid feeling flustered or wishy-washy in the heat of the moment. Remember, put yourself first!

Another tip I share with my patients is this: Write down your goals and values. Knowing your values and setting specific goals that support them is critically important. These values and goals may have nothing to do with sex—maybe you want to save the world from climate change by discovering a green fuel or to become a novelist or a doctor or the first woman president. Whatever your big goals are, when you write them down and outline the steps to get there, you may realize that having sex at a young age (and therefore risking pregnancy or a life-changing sexually transmitted infection) doesn't fit in with your grand scheme.

I also recommend making a pros and cons list about the potential good and bad consequences of losing your virginity. Seeing that list in black and white might clarify some issues for you. If the negatives outweigh the positives, you probably shouldn't do it.

Finally, realize that your success or failure rests largely with you—and *only* you. This is true for love, for life goals, and for your choices about sexual activity. Even though you might not be a legal adult, as a teenager you have quite a bit of power and autonomy. Your parents may still call a lot of the shots, but your life is largely in your hands. You have the freedom to decide how to behave, what you'll do, and what you won't do. In almost all cases, no one can really force you to do something you don't want to do. The downside of all this power is that you're responsible for your own successes or failures. Making mistakes is part of growing up, and many can become powerful learning experiences. Just try not to make the same mistakes over and over again. This is part of what determines a person's ultimate success: It's not just where you finish that matters, it's also how far you've come!

READY-MADE RESPONSES

Honesty is definitely the best policy when it comes to not having sex. If you don't want to and you're not ready, you shouldn't have to explain yourself. Just tell your boyfriend clearly where you draw the line. He should respect that. If he doesn't, you should dump him and find someone who listens to you.

But I'm a realist. I know things don't always seem quite so simple in the heat of the moment. Here are some things my patients have told their boyfriends—some the straightforward truth . . . some not so much.

1. "I've decided not to have sex until I'm eighteen. If we're still dating then, maybe I'll think about it."
2. "There's no way to be 100 percent sure I won't get pregnant or get an STI, and there's no way I'm taking even a small risk."
3. "I'm not ready to have sex. I know it's not right for me yet, and if you don't respect that, I'll date someone else."
4. "My parents promised me a car if I'm still a virgin when I graduate."
5. "I can't have sex because I can't use condoms—I'm allergic to latex."

DR. ASHTON'S WHY-WAIT FAQs

When we have the wait-till-eighteen talk, most of my patients have similar questions. Here's what I tell them:

THEY ASK:	I SAY:
Why wait?	It's important for your health—mind and body.
Does it really matter?	Yes! The younger you are when you start having sex, the worse it is for your health.
What's the worst that could happen?	You could get a horrible infection and/or get pregnant and your life might never be the same again.
How do I wait?	Have your responses ready and outline your goals.

DR. ASHTON'S WAIT-TILL-EIGHTEEN PLAYLIST

- Wait as long as possible for sex—at least until eighteen. The longer you wait for sex, the better for your lifetime health.
- If you want to engage in adult behavior, you have to accept adult responsibilities. If you have sex, you have to be ready to see a gynecologist, have a pelvic exam, use (and pay for) two kinds of contraception (condoms and a backup method like the pill), buy condoms at the drugstore, get screened for sexually transmitted infections, and engage in awkward conversations about all this with your boyfriend.
- You don't have to have sex—there are plenty of other things you and your boyfriend can do. (But remember—you can get herpes, genital warts, and all other STIs from oral sex, so use condoms even then.)
- Someday you'll have sex. But that's not a box you need to check now. You can wait as long as you want—the longer, the better, from a medical point of view.

SURVIVING SEX ED

If your sex ed class is anything like mine was, it's *torture*. First, mine was taught by the gym teachers, not by nurses or medical professionals. Second, it was a coed class. Trust me when I say that sitting next to the guy you have a crush on while hearing about periods and erections is an embarrassing agony you do *not* want to live through.

Horrible as it was, what's even *more* horrifying is that in the past twenty or thirty years, hardly anything has changed in the way sex ed is taught (except that now they sometimes they call it "reproductive health" instead of sex ed, because it sounds less scandalous). But come on! TV, movies, magazines, and just daily life expose young people to much more sexual content today than ever. On TV alone you're exposed to twice as much sexual content as teens were just a decade ago. With teens getting so many more messages about sex and knowing so much more than they used to, you'd think sex ed would be more sophisticated, too. But sex ed has hardly changed a bit.

I learned this the hard way, when I started to explain things like STIs and contraception to my patients, figuring they already knew all about this stuff. "I'm sure this is nothing new to you," I'd say, "but you do realize you can get herpes from oral sex, right?" Under other circumstances their shocked, dismayed, and horrified expressions might have been pretty funny. But this was too important to laugh at. So I'd start from scratch with my explanation.

I usually find the same shock and dismay when I go into schools to talk about STIs and contraception. Even the best schools don't always cover all the bases. When I spoke at one of the top high schools in my state of New Jersey, the students were appalled to learn how easy it is to get herpes and that even virgins can get it. Sex ed curriculum varies across the country, so there's no way to know whether your school is going to cover everything you really need to know.

Why don't our schools do a better job? Partly because some adults just aren't comfortable talking with teens about these issues. Many adults fear that explaining things to teens will send them off on a wild quest for non-stop sex and drugs. But, actually, the research shows the opposite is true. Teens who learn accurate, factual information about sex and other high-risk behaviors are much more likely *not* to engage in early sexual activity. So read, listen, ask, and talk. The more info you have, the better.

Another reason U.S. schools fall down on the job of teaching sex ed is that most teachers aren't trained in the subject. Studies show that nationally 18 percent of all sex ed teachers have received no formal training in that subject.[25] The numbers are even higher in some states. In Illinois, for example, one in three sex ed teachers has not been formally trained in how to teach that subject.[26] Nationally, four in ten sex ed teachers either don't teach their students about contraception at all or teach that contraception doesn't work![27] Yikes!

Some schools and states just don't have the budget to fund training, so many teachers step into the sex ed classroom with no more preparation than a preapproved curriculum and a meeting with a principal or administrator. That'd be like me teaching a bunch of culinary students to make soufflé—when I can barely boil water.

To make matters worse, this isn't any old subject—it's one that some adults are positively allergic to. These poor teachers aren't doctors or nurses. Even if they were, they still might be very uncomfortable (even my own mom and dad—a doctor and a nurse—could barely bring themselves to talk to me openly about sex!). Your teacher might feel perfectly fine talking about abstinence but not so comfortable explaining how to use a condom. So your class might not get the best instruction on condom use.

Finally, learning about sex ed is very different from learning geometry. There's no one answer, no right way to communicate the facts. There are many different schools of thought about what should be taught and how. Many things, from state standards to teachers' personal values to parental input and teaching resources, can affect what you learn. So take responsibility and make sure you're getting the facts you need by reviewing the survey in the box below. Remember—knowledge is power!

POP QUIZ: HAS YOUR SEX ED CLASS (OR HEALTH CLASS) COVERED THIS?

If your sex ed class doesn't cover all the topics in the list below, ask your pediatrician, gynecologist, or parents to fill in the gaps. You owe it to your future health.

☐ Information on puberty and reproduction
☐ Information on STIs, HIV, and AIDS
☐ Information about abstinence and contraception (including how to put on a condom)
☐ Sexual violence and gender issues
☐ Relationships (family and sexual)

- ☐ Effects of smoking, drinking, and drug use
- ☐ Communication and behavioral and decision-making skills
- ☐ Issues of self-esteem and body image

? DID YOU KNOW?
Your Parents Have Some Good Stories

Your parents may not be as dumb as you think. Try asking them how old they were when they started having sex. Or if they regretted it. Or if they had any funny or memorable stories or words of wisdom for you. You may be surprised at what you learn—and your parents might actually be relieved that you want to talk openly about sex.

ONE MORE REASON TO POSTPONE SEX

Ever hear the old saying that bad things happen in threes? Sexual activity at a young age is no exception. Statistics show that teens who are sexually active are also at higher risk for two more risky activities—smoking and the use of illegal substances, including alcohol. All these behaviors are harmful in and of themselves, but they also tend to lead to unsafe situations—including abuse, rape, and other sexual violence. We've all heard the horrible stories about teens killed in drunk driving accidents or who were abducted, raped, or murdered. Avoiding sex before age eighteen may help you steer clear of other risky behaviors and keep you from becoming a tragic statistic.

DID YOU KNOW?
Teen Girls Face the Highest Risk of Sexual Violence

Sexual violence—be it stranger rape, date rape, or abuse by a family member or other acquaintance—is never, *ever* the victim's fault. It's a violent crime that has absolutely nothing to do with what the victim wore, said, or did. Sadly, these terrible acts of violence happen more often to teen girls than any other group of people. If you're a victim of sexual violence (defined as any physical or verbal act that's sexual in nature and violates your trust and/or your safety), please know that this is *not your fault.* Many victims of sexual violence feel guilty and ashamed and have trouble trusting people. You deserve help. Many communities have rape crisis centers with twenty-four-hour hotlines, and any teen being abused can contact the twenty-four-hour National Child Abuse Hotline for help: 1-800-422-4453. For more information, visit www.childhelp.org.

MORE FACTS ABOUT SEXUAL VIOLENCE[28]

- A woman is four times more likely to be raped by someone she knows than by a stranger.
- Women ages fourteen to seventeen represent an estimated 38 percent of those victimized by date rape.
- Dating violence affects at least one in ten teen couples.
- More than half of high school boys and 42 percent of high school girls believe there are times when it is "acceptable for a male to hold a female down and physically force her to engage in intercourse." But let me be very clear: It is, in fact,

NEVER acceptable for anyone to force you to have intercourse. Not physically. Not emotionally. No one has the right to make you do anything you don't want to do.

NO REGRETS

After reading all this, I hope you'll agree there are very, very good medical reasons to postpone having sex. But in the end it comes down to this: Don't you want your first time to be healthy, happy, and fun—and not something you cringe about twenty years from now? The longer you wait, the more likely it is you'll get your wish and have no regrets. That's what happened with my patient Sarah. And that's what I want for you, too. No regrets!

CHAPTER 9

NEVER TELL YOUR BOYFRIEND YOU'RE ON THE PILL

(and Other Rules for a Healthy Sex Life)

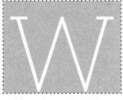hen it comes to having the "big talk" about sex, my parents sort of missed the boat. Actually, they never even bought a ticket.

For my mom's part, she spoke in code. What she *meant* was, "Tell me when you're having sex."

What she *said* (repeatedly) was, "Just let me know when you need to see the gynecologist."

Every single time she uttered this phrase, I wanted to yell, "Mom! Why can't you just say the word? SEX!" And . . . hello? She was a *nurse*! (I still appreciated her efforts, however. Some parents never say anything at all to their children about sex.)

If she had trouble talking about sex, imagine how hard it is for parents who don't deal with the human body and all its quirks day in and day out.

My father, a doctor, was more the strong, silent type when it came to sex. What he *did* say has stayed with me until this day. The sum total of his big sex talk with me was this: "Never do anything you don't want to do." Now, this is great advice, and I'll tell you why later. I'm proud of him for even bringing up the topic with me. But . . . just one sentence? From a doctor? Please!

Of course, most of the time my patients' parents aren't doctors. And usually they have no idea how to bring up sex without embarrassing you and themselves. In fact, these days my patients are often way more relaxed bringing up the subject with their parents than vice versa.

Even when the parents of my patients do bite the bullet and talk about sex and contraception, their information often isn't up to date. It's usually been a while since they brushed up on the topic. So to make sure you've gotten all the info, I'm going to review everything you need to know to have a healthy, happy sex life. I'm fervently hoping that you won't need this until *after* you turn eighteen (and I encourage you to read the last chapter again anytime you're feeling wishy-washy on that subject). But in any case, when you do start having sex, it's my job to guide you in doing it safely. Here's what I tell my sexually active patients.

DR. ASHTON'S FIVE SIMPLE RULES FOR A HEALTHY SEX LIFE

1. Never tell your boyfriend you're on the pill.

Yes, you heard me right. I'm telling you to lie to your boyfriend. Because, I promise you, if he knows you're on the pill or another form of birth control, he won't use a condom every time. And you always need to use two forms of birth control—one to prevent pregnancy (see my list of options at the end of this chapter), plus condoms to avoid sexually transmitted infections.

Remember, it only takes *one time* to get an STI. My patient Julia learned this the hard way. After a very sheltered upbringing, she went to college, where she went a little wild. She started drinking and partying—and the very first guy she slept with gave her chlamydia (read all about this lovely disease in chapter 10).

So, as I advise all my patients, don't tell your boyfriend you're on the pill or other birth control. If he asks why you're not, tell him you get migraines or you have a clotting disorder, so you can't take birth control hormones. Yeah, it's a white lie. So what? What he doesn't know won't hurt him. And it *can* help you—*a lot.*

2. Tell your mother (or father) when you're sexually active.

I urge my patients to tell their parents when they start having sex. Parents might not be thrilled, but it's their job to know about anything that could affect your health and safety. And, awkward as it is, most moms want to know on some level. Given how hard it is for them to bring up the topic, parents may actually be relieved when you tell them.

3. If you want to engage in adult behaviors, you need to act like an adult.

Sex is an adult behavior that requires other adult behaviors—many of which aren't all that fun. Those include seeing a gynecologist regularly—complete with stirrups, speculum, and regular pelvic exams. It also means being willing to start awkward conversations, like talking with your boyfriend about STIs and birth control and letting your parents know what's happening.

4. Never do anything you don't want to do.

Thanks, Dad! This is still one of the very best pieces of sexual advice I've ever heard. The sad fact is that one in four women will be abused at some time during her life.[29] So I want you to know right now that no one has the right to ever hurt you or force you into sexual activities you don't want. If it happens, I want you to tell your doctor, your parents, or someone else you trust right away. Don't feel bad or ashamed—just get checked out to make sure you're OK.

This rule applies to emotional abuse, too. Once, when I was in college, I was crying to my brother about how my boyfriend had treated me badly. I wanted to give him another shot. "Jen," said my brother, "*no one deserves a second shot with you.*" I feel the same way about you. Nobody has the right to hurt you and nobody who does hurt you deserves a second shot. You're too good for that.

If you've been sexually abused or mistreated, please know it's not your fault—and get some help and support. See chapter 8 for resources.

5. Don't date guys more than a year older than you are.

This relates back to Rule Number 4: Never do anything you don't want to do. Boyfriends who are significantly older than you will have more experience and will pressure you to go further—sometimes *much* further.

I'll never forget Lisa, a model-gorgeous fifteen-year-old. She and her mother came to see me because Lisa thought she might be pregnant by her twenty-five-year-old boyfriend. She was. She decided to end the pregnancy, but she didn't break it off with the guy. (Note that a grown man having sex with a fifteen-year-old is not only deeply disturbing, but it's *against the law*.) Within two years he'd given her chlamydia. I was very concerned about her health and worried about her having a relationship with a man ten years older than she was.

"You know," I said to her carefully, "sometimes . . . actually, more often than not . . . older guys will put younger girls in risky situations." With that she broke into tears. Before the visit was over, she told me he'd asked her to have sex with his friends—and she'd done it, at least once. He'd also persuaded her to try pot, cocaine, and ecstasy. I told Lisa I thought she was in danger and that these patterns often lead to physical abuse, even death. No sooner did those words cross my lips than this beautiful, scared teenager pulled up the legs on her sweatpants to reveal huge, shocking bruises. Her boyfriend had hit her with a baseball bat.

All of this, in my professional opinion, definitely qualified for breaching the doctor-patient confidentiality agreement. I felt her life was literally in danger. I immediately brought her mom into my office for a major intervention and helped Lisa and her mother find a residential treatment program that helps teens in trouble.

Lisa's now on a much healthier path. When I saw her recently for a checkup, she gave me a huge hug and told me she'd been addicted to drugs and alcohol back then. But now she'd been sober for more than two years. At the end of our visit, she hugged me again. With tears rolling down her face, she said, "You saved my life, Dr. Ashton." Lisa had been very close to becoming one of those statistics we hear about on the evening news.

Of course, not all older guys will turn out to be like the man who abused Lisa. But dating boys your own age will help keep you in control of the situation Plus, they'll probably have a level of sexual experience that is closer to your own.

GAY TEENS

Nationally, 2 to 4 percent of teen girls identify themselves as lesbians. When patients tell me that they're attracted to girls, I share with them two key medical facts.

- You can still get STIs even if you're not having vaginal intercourse.
- Beware of medical discrimination against lesbians.

Many gynecologists assume that if a woman isn't having vaginal sex with a man, she should be treated medically like a virgin. That's not true. I urge my gay patients to be vigilant about their health and make sure they always receive the care they need, including Pap smears and regular testing for STIs.

THE NEW BASICS OF BIRTH CONTROL

If you remember nothing else in this book, remember this: **If you don't use birth control, you are very likely to get pregnant.**

Every year 85 percent of women who have sex without using birth control get pregnant, according to Planned Parenthood. This is like playing Russian roulette. It's not cool and it's very dangerous. If you have sex, you need to use two forms of birth control—a condom and a backup method like the pill, since condoms fail to prevent pregnancy 15 percent of the time.[30]

 DID YOU KNOW?
Unintended Pregnancies Happen All the Time

Even though the rate of teen pregnancies has been on the decline in recent years (until they increased slightly between 2005 and 2006), it's still much too high. Some 750,000 girls ages fifteen to nineteen get pregnant every year.[31] About 34 percent choose to terminate the pregnancy.[32] Some teens keep their babies; others give them up for adoption. Whatever direction they take, their high school years will never be the same and their choices will have long-term consequences.

 DR. ASHTON'S SAFE SEX PLAYLIST

- *Always* use two forms of birth control . . . unless you *want* to get pregnant or catch an STI.
- Never ever have sex without a condom.
- Know that you can get herpes and any other STI from oral sex.
- Just because you lose your virginity doesn't mean you have to sleep with every boyfriend in your future. Keep your lifetime number low to stay healthy.

? TRUE OR FALSE?

The pill can lead to infertility over time.

> **FALSE**. The pill does not lead to infertility.

You should give your body a break from the pill from time to time.

> **FALSE**. Nope, no breaks necessary. Going off the pill for a while doesn't help your body in any way.

Hormones, including the pill, cause cancer.

> **FALSE**. Conclusive studies show that the birth control pill does not cause cancer. In fact, it decreases the risk of ovarian and uterine cancer by up to 50 percent.

Teens have two birth control options: condoms or the pill.

> **FALSE**. There are more than half a dozen birth control options for teen girls, including the Ring and the IUD. (See the birth control briefing, below.) But remember—condoms are the only contraceptive that protects against STIs.

The pill causes headaches and weight gain.

> **FALSE**. Although versions of the pill in the 1970s sometimes had side effects like headaches and weight gain, those happen less frequently with today's pills, which include lower doses of hormones.

> *You have to have a Pap smear when you go to the ob-gyn.*
>
> **FALSE**. Girls don't need their first Pap smear until age twenty-one if they haven't had sex. But they should have one within three years after becoming sexually active.
>
> *Condoms protect against all sexually transmitted infections.*
>
> **FALSE**. Condoms provide only partial protection. For example, HPV, the virus that causes genital warts, is transferred by skin-to-skin contact. Since condoms don't cover every skin surface, they don't protect against HPV.

BIRTH CONTROL BRIEFING

Don't expect to learn all you need to know about birth control in school. Many schools provide no instruction in birth control methods except for abstinence.

It's a shame, because there are more birth control options than ever, many newly approved for teens. Of course, condoms are still the only way to prevent most STIs. But you need to use two birth control methods—condoms *and* a backup method to prevent pregnancy. (I know, I'm repeating myself . . . but I don't want you to get pregnant or end up with an STI.)

Why? Because condoms have a 15 percent failure rate with typical use—much higher than the failure rate of other methods, like the pill.

One of my patients, Susan, learned this the hard way. While she was away at college she got pregnant and had a termination procedure at a Planned Parenthood near her school. As if that weren't enough, she also got chlamydia and HPV from her steady boyfriend—a triple whammy. When she came home for a checkup, I asked what had happened.

"I don't know," she said. "We used condoms every single time. And I never saw one that looked broken or torn." It was a perfect example of the 15 percent failure rule: You might not even notice when a condom is leaking or torn. Remember Susan when you're thinking that safe sex (sex with condoms) has no risks. The best way to be safe is to avoid sex; the second best way is to be discriminating and always use two forms of birth control.

BIRTH CONTROL MENU[33]

Here's a guide to your choices.

Condoms

The *only* method of contraception that prevents the spread of sexually transmitted infections. I tell my patients never to have sex without a condom. But even condoms have a 15 percent failure rate with typical use. ("Typical use" refers to the fact that they may rip, slip off, etc.) You absolutely must use a backup method (just don't tell your boyfriend about it or he'll think it's OK to skip the condom).

Unfortunately, despite all the media campaigns and educational efforts to promote condom use, only 62 percent of high school students who have had sex say they used a condom the last time they had intercourse. That number is much too low. It needs to be 100 percent. Do your part: Always use condoms.

FIVE MORE REASONS TO LOVE CONDOMS

1. They're cheap.
2. They're easy to get at any drugstore.
3. No prescription needed: Anyone can buy them.

4. Minors can buy them.
5. Did I mention that they're the *only way* to avoid STIs?

Hormonal Methods

Most other contraceptive methods involve hormones, delivered through a pill, patch, shot, or other method. No hormonal method protects against STIs. (But . . . they do clear up acne!) As you consider hormonal options, also look back at chapter 3, on periods, where I talk about myths regarding the pill.

Oral Contraceptives ("The Pill")

Oral contraceptives usually are a combination of two hormones—estrogen and progestin. Working together they prevent ovulation, thin the uterine lining, and thicken cervical mucus. The progestin-only "mini-pill" doesn't include estrogen but needs to be taken at *exactly* the same time each day, which can be tough for teens.

How well does it work? It's 99.7 percent effective with perfect use: Only one in a thousand women taking their pill every single day without fail would become pregnant. With typical use (that is, forgetting to take a pill now and then), the pill is 92 percent effective. This means that eight in one hundred women will get pregnant on the pill. (Trust me, it really happens: I've delivered babies conceived this way.)

PROS:
- Safe (Except for women over thirty-five who smoke or who have classic migraines with visual disturbances before the headaches start. The pill is not recommended for these women due to an increased risk of blood clots.)

- Cuts the risk of ovarian and uterine cancer by half
- The most popular method of contraception among teens

CONS:
- You need a prescription.
- It doesn't protect against STIs.
- You have to take your pill every day.
- It's associated with an increased rate of cervical cancer (although experts think this increased risk comes from not using condoms and therefore contracting HPV, which is linked to cervical cancer).
- It can be expensive.

BAD CHEMISTRY

Certain medications can affect the pill, making it less effective. If you're taking any of the following, it's even more important that you use a second method of birth control—or you may end up pregnant despite your faithful pill popping.

- Seizure medication
- St. John's wort
- The antibiotic Rifampin, which is used to treat tuberculosis
- Anti-HIV drugs

? TRUE OR FALSE?

Teens need a full gynecological exam, including a pelvic exam, before starting on the pill.

FALSE. It's a good idea but it's not a must.

Yep, it's true—your pediatrician can write your birth control prescription. Your pediatrician can also answer your questions about sex and guide you on safe practices. Of course, I think it's a great idea to have your own gynecologist before you start having sex, but I know that's not always possible. And not having a gynecologist is no excuse for getting pregnant!

The Ring

Approved in 2001, the Ring is a soft, flexible silicone ring that releases estrogen and progestin and carries about the same low risks as the pill. You remove it after three weeks, then insert a new one a week later. A nice feature of the Ring is that it keeps your hormone levels slightly lower than even the lowest-dose pill. Also, since the medication is absorbed via the vagina, the hormones don't have to be processed by your liver the way they do with the oral pill. I don't have many patients using the Ring, because most don't like the idea of inserting something in their vaginas (funny, isn't it?). My teen patients who do use the Ring like the fact that they don't have to remember to take a pills every day—and that it's a lot easier to hide than a pill container.

How well does it work? It is assumed to be as effective or even more effective than the pill. It's more than 99 percent effective with perfect use in adult women and 92 percent effective with typical use.

PROS:
- Safe (same low risks as the pill)
- Convenient—you only have to think about it twice a month (once when you take it out, once when you put a new one in)

177

CONS:
- Hasn't been formally studied in teens
- Might cause vaginal discharge or discomfort
- Doesn't protect against STIs
- Can slip out . . . but still works if replaced within three hours

The Patch

This is a skin-colored patch, worn on the stomach, back, arm, or buttocks, that releases estrogen and progestin.

How well does it work? It's 99 percent effective with perfect use; 92 percent with typical use.

PROS:
- Safe
- Convenient (change it once a week for three weeks, then leave it off for a week)
- Discreet

CONS:
- No protection against STIs
- Might have a higher failure rate for women weighing more than 198 pounds
- In 2005 the FDA required the manufacturer to warn on the label that women are exposed to 60 percent more estrogen than with most forms of the pill—though it's not clear that the extra estrogen poses extra risk. This has been the subject of much debate, and most doctors believe it to deliver a much lower dose of estrogen.
- Carries a slightly higher risk of blood clots than the pill. But that risk is still very small: three or four out of ten thousand instead of one out of ten thousand.

The Shot

Depo-Provera injections, which contain progestin only, are given by a doctor every three months. This injection has been available since 1992 and is well studied in teens. However, I do not prescribe Depo-Provera for my patients and don't recommend it for teens because it carries a risk of osteoporosis later in life.

How well does it work? It's 97 percent effective. Because the shot is given by a doctor, there's no risk of imperfect use unless you don't show up for your shot.

PROS:

- No estrogen-related side effects
- Good if you just can't remember to take a pill daily or change a patch or ring weekly or monthly

CONS:

- You may gain about fifteen pounds (one common side effect, and a big deterrent for my patients!) and it might cause acne and headaches.
- Requires shots every three months
- Injected hormones can lead to a temporary thinning of the bones, so most women shouldn't use the method for longer than two years. The shot carries an FDA warning against its increased risk of osteoporosis.
- Potential for heavy bleeding and irregular spotting

The IUD

This small, T-shaped plastic device inserted by a doctor in the uterus is now available for teens. The IUD works by preventing fertilization and implantation. Although some IUDs were taken off the market back in the 1970s and 1980s, in recent years IUDs have become one of the most popular types of reversible birth control worldwide. One type, Mirena, releases progesterone and prevents pregnancy for five years. The other type, Para-Gard, contains copper, which helps prevent fertilization, and can be left in place for ten years.

A generation ago old-school doctors wouldn't even consider using an IUD for a teenager (or even for an unmarried woman). That's because the devices available back then had a high risk of causing a uterine or pelvic infection, which could affect your fertility. Back then the strings attached to the little IUD device were made of a material that was super-easy for bacteria to grab onto and climb up into the uterus, where they caused infections. Today those strings are made of a different material, and the bacteria slip off more easily. The risk of pelvic infection still exists, but it's much lower than it used to be—so low that gynecologists who treat a lot of adolescents now feel comfortable prescribing IUDs even for teens. This isn't the right choice for every teenager, but it's another option—as long as you understand that with this device in your uterus practicing safe sex is even more critically important!

How well does it work? It's 99 percent effective with typical use.

PROS:
- Convenient
- No pills to take or rings or patches to change
- One particular brand (Mirena) can cause lighter menstrual flows.

CONS:
- Must be inserted by a physician
- Spotting between periods is common for the first few months
- One brand (ParaGard) can increase menstrual flow and, in some cases, lead to anemia
- Cramps or backaches
- Can slip out or puncture the wall of the uterus, though this usually doesn't happen—the risk is 2 to 10 percent.
- Can cause infection—this is rare (especially after the first three weeks after insertion) but possible, especially if patient has been exposed to chlamydia or gonorrhea.

The Sponge

This is a small polyurethane sponge treated with spermicide. You insert the sponge up to thirty hours before you have sex and remove it within thirty hours after. After being off the market for years, the Today Sponge returned in 2005.

How well does it work? Not well. It's only 85 percent effective with perfect use. With typical use, thirty out of one hundred women will get pregnant while using the sponge. That's really high!

PROS:

- Convenient: Can be carried in a purse and inserted up to thirty hours before intercourse
- Available over the counter

CONS:

- No protection against sexually transmitted diseases
- Far less effective than other methods
- Should not be used during menstruation
- Can be difficult to insert properly and/or remove

Implanon

In 2006 the FDA approved Implanon, a tiny rod inserted under the skin of the upper arm that releases progestin. Implanon can safely be used in teens and can stay in place for up to three years.

How well does it work? It's almost 100 percent effective.

PROS:

- Convenient—no effort required
- Helps acne—59 percent of women in clinical trials who had acne said it lessened or went away after they started using Implanon.

CONS:

- Must be inserted and removed by a physician
- Expensive
- Can cause irregular bleeding (although many women stop having their periods at all)

The Female Condom

OK, I admit it. I've never had a single patient who has used the female condom. But you should know it's an option. It's basically a latex pouch inserted into the vagina before sex. Like traditional condoms, it provides a roadblock that (theoretically) sperm can't penetrate. It does provide some measure of protection against STIs. Like condoms, it's not considered highly effective for birth control: As many as fifteen out of one hundred times the female condom will fail, leading to pregnancy or STIs. Important note: You can't use both a female condom and a traditional condom at the same time. You have to use just one or the other.

PROS:

- Relatively cheap
- Easy to get
- Can reduce the chance of pregnancy and STIs

CONS:

- Difficult and awkward to use
- More expensive than male condoms
- It makes noise!

Spermicides

Sounds like pesticides, right? Same idea—spermicides kill sperm. Most contain the chemical nonoxynol-9. You apply them to your vagina in various ways: foams, gels, films, or suppositories/inserts. Spermicides must be used in conjunction with condoms—just using spermicide alone won't protect you from STIs and provides only some protection against pregnancy.

PROS:

- When used with condoms, very effective at contraception and reducing STIs
- Cheap
- Easily available
- No prescription needed

CONS:

- Nonoxynol-9 can irritate the vagina.
- There's no guarantee that all sperm will be blocked or killed with nonoxynol-9 and condoms—and it only takes ONE little sperm to get you pregnant.
- Some studies suggest nonoxynol-9 can increase the chances of getting HIV due to irritation of the vagina.

NOT FOR TEENS: DON'T TRY THESE

Diaphragms, cervical caps, and shields are not good options for teens (or adults for that matter). These are all "barriers" inserted into the vagina. Unfortunately, they have a high failure rate—20 percent with a diaphragm, 40 percent with a cap. Plus, if a cap is left in for more than two days, there's a higher risk of toxic shock syndrome—a potentially life-threatening infection. These methods require precise measurement and fitting by a doctor to make sure you get the right size. Last but definitely not least, most teenagers simply don't want to insert stuff into their vaginas. Because of all these problems, I don't even recommend these for my adult patients.

GREAT WAYS TO GET PREGNANT: METHODS THAT DON'T WORK

Here are a couple of things that **just don't work** (unless, that is, you're *trying* to get pregnant):

1. The so-called **rhythm method**, where you count the days of your cycle and avoid sex during and after ovulation. **The rhythm method is a disastrous choice for teens.** Until you're in your twenties, your cycles are not regular enough to predict ovulation with any accuracy. Even for adult women this method has a 15 to 30 percent failure rate.

2. **Withdrawal**, where the man withdraws his penis from the vagina before he ejaculates. Not only does this method require enormous self-control—not something teen boys are famous for—but it also doesn't work. Typically, withdrawal has a failure rate of about 20 to 30 percent. That's because the fluid released before ejaculation can contain sperm, which can swim into the vagina from the vulva.

LIP SERVICE: SAFE ORAL SEX

So by now you're probably thinking, "How many more times is Dr. Ashton going to tell me that you can get an STI from oral sex? I understand, OK?!? So what am I supposed to do about it? Not have oral sex?"

Actually, that's not a bad idea for your health, especially if you're under eighteen. But let's be realistic. The fact is, you *can* have safe oral sex. It's simple. If you're performing oral sex on your boyfriend, make him wear a condom. And if he's the performer, he should use a dental dam—basically a small, thin piece of latex that acts as a barrier to bodily fluids, reducing STI transmission. The partner who's giving oral sex holds the dam against the body part in question, then sets to work. Some people recommend using a water-based lubricant for comfort. Don't use an oil-based lubricant or lotion, since it can break down the latex. Be sure to use just one side of the dam and don't reuse it on another body part: There's no recycling here.

EMERGENCY CONTRACEPTION: WHAT TO DO IF THE CONDOM BREAKS

Everybody goofs sometimes. If you've just had sex without birth control or if the condom broke, it's not too late to help prevent pregnancy. Emergency contraception is available over the counter for women ages eighteen and over. Currently girls younger than eighteen need a prescription for the morning-after pill, but soon it may be available to them over the counter.

The most common emergency contraception, approved since 1999, is called Plan B. Plan B and similar medications prevent conception from taking place. It does not cause abortions. In fact, emergency contraception actually prevents an estimated 50,000 abortions from taking place each year.

Plan B contains progestin in two pills. You take the first dose within seventy-two hours of unprotected sex. You take the second twelve hours later. (Alternatively, you can take both pills at the same time.) It does cause irregular bleeding after you take it. And since it doesn't always work, you should take pregnancy tests two and four weeks after taking EC. You also need to get tested for STIs: The same sperm that can get you pregnant might carry infections and diseases.

The sooner you take Plan B, the better it will work. If you take it within twenty-four hours, it's 90 percent effective, meaning you probably won't get pregnant. But if you use it three days later, it's only 75 percent effective. And it's just 60 percent effective if you take it five days later.

WARNING: Emergency contraception should NOT count as one of your two birth control methods! It's not perfect by any means. Unfortunately, not everyone gets that message. One new patient told me she'd already used emergency contraception, which she'd obtained at a clinic, three times and admitted she hadn't used any other form of birth control. In other words, emergency contraception was her *only* contraception.

"That's not the right way to use emergency contraception," I told her. "If that's your only method, it's only a matter of time until you get pregnant—and probably pick up a sexually transmitted infection, too." She asked me for a prescription for the pill, which I gladly gave her.

MORE READY-MADE EXCUSES

Remember in the last chapter I suggested you plan ahead about what you'll say to avoid having sex? It's also a great idea to practice a few handy excuses when you're trying to be safe about sex. Again, honesty is always the best policy and always the route I recommend. But if that absolutely won't work for you, I've included a few other ideas that my patients have used with great success:

- Getting an STI would really mess up both our lives. Either we use condoms or we don't have sex. Better safe than sorry.
- "My doctor says I can't take birth control pills because I get mi-

graines (or because I have a blood clotting disorder). So we have to use condoms."

- "I think I'm getting a cold sore. We should be extra-safe so you don't get one, too—especially down there."
- "I've got my period."

Remember—you've (hopefully) waited a long time to have sex. Make it worth the wait by doing everything in your power to guarantee yourself a safe, happy experience that you'll enjoy remembering later on.

CHAPTER 10

THE HUMAN PYRAMID SCHEME

Avoiding the Big Three Sexually Transmitted Infections

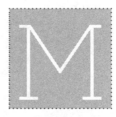y patient Shannon was home from college recently and dropped in for a routine visit. For the past ten months she'd been dating Jeff, her first serious boyfriend. They'd started having sex a few months earlier. He was her first, and vice versa. What could be more romantic—or more healthy?

I did a pelvic exam that included a routine test for chlamydia, a very common sexually transmitted infection. Imagine Shannon's surprise when I called and told her the results.

"So, Shannon, I have some bad news," I said. "Your tests came back positive for chlamydia."

"That can't be right," she said. "The lab must have messed up. Jeff and I haven't ever slept with other people."

The lab wasn't wrong, and it didn't take a CSI team to figure out what happened. Jeff had cheated on her. When Shannon confronted him, he admitted he'd slept with another girl—just once, he swore—during a family vacation to Florida. Instead of an ugly tourist T-shirt, he brought her back chlamydia. Nothing says "I love you" quite like a sexually transmitted infection.

Unfortunately, Shannon learned the hard way that contraception and safe sex are two different things. She was on the pill, which reduced her chances of pregnancy. But she *didn't* always practice safe sex—that is, sex with a condom. Intellectually she knew she needed to use the pill *and* condoms, every time. But emotionally she felt that she could cheat on the condom part, since she and Jeff were (supposedly) monogamous. Unfortunately, it only took one slip (as far we know) to infect Jeff and then Shannon.

Shannon might not have been so smart about condoms, but she *was* smart to see a gynecologist regularly. Chlamydia is easy to treat if you catch it early. When I told her simple antibiotics would clear it up, Shannon felt a little better—about the physical stuff, that is.

The emotional hurt is still healing.

THE BIG THREE: CHLAMYDIA, HPV, AND HERPES

Shannon's not exactly the only girl to receive an unwanted souvenir from her partner's sexual adventures. More than 1.1 million people got chlamydia in 2007.[34] The HPV virus, which causes genital warts, is even more common—24.5 percent of girls ages fourteen to nineteen have this virus, and 44.8 percent of women twenty to twenty-four have it.[35] Up to 50 percent of sexually active adults will have HPV at some point in their lives.[36] And don't forget genital herpes, carried by a whopping one in five people in the United States.[37]

Chlamydia, HPV, and herpes are just three of many sexually transmitted infections, none of which you want (especially after you see the pictures in the medical textbooks . . .). But they're the three I see most often in my teenage patients. In fact, they're so common I call them the "infection trifecta." Learning the basics of the Big Three should tell you all you need to know to avoid every sexually transmitted infection (STI).

> ## STI: THE BOTTOM LINE
>
> Feel like skipping this chapter? Just read this: **Never, ever, ever have sex without a condom** until you're married or with a life partner. End of story.

THE HUMAN PYRAMID SCHEME: HOW STIs WORK

Every now and then you read about somebody going to jail for running a pyramid scheme: It's a scam where you persuade a couple of people to give you money . . . then they persuade a few others to give them money . . . and it all passes up the pyramid. The person at the top wins. The ones at the bottom lose big-time.

With sexually transmitted infections, *everybody* in the pyramid loses. Meaning that when you sleep with someone, you're exposing yourself to everyone they have ever slept with. And everyone *those* people have ever slept with. And so on.

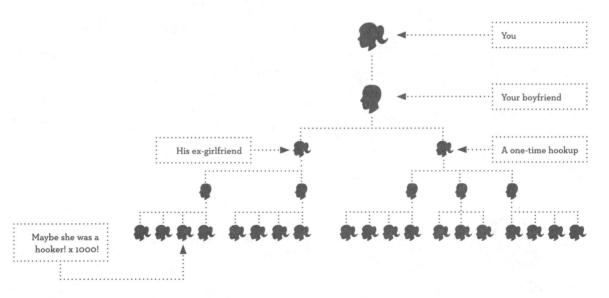

WHY YOU DON'T WANT AN STI

Trust me, you do not want an STI. Come on by my office sometime and I'll show you the pictures. *Blech.* Here are a few more reasons.

- You might end up infertile. Infections like chlamydia and gonorrhea can scar your fallopian tubes and lead to infertility. OK, right now avoiding babies sounds good. In fact, that's your goal. But you won't want the stress and heartbreak of infertility when you're ready to start a family.
- You might have serious health problems for *the rest of your life.* With herpes, for instance, you'll get painful sores on your genitals from time to time until you die.
- There's still a social stigma against STIs, even though they're incredibly common: After all, would *you* deliberately choose to hook up with someone with herpes? (Of course, it's a whole different story when you really fall in love with someone you want to marry. I never heard of anyone calling off an engagement due to herpes, although I'm sure it must happen . . .)

When I was a kid, the term "VD" (see above) was used to refer to all sexually transmitted diseases, without much distinction between them. Today teens know more about specific infections: Some of my patients can rattle off all the proper medical names and even rank the relative desirability of each. ("You might have chlamydia, but at least you don't have syphilis!") You probably also know you can pick up an infection with just *one single isolated act of sexual contact*—including oral sex or genital contact without penetration. You don't have to be easy, sleazy, or skanky to get one—just unlucky and maybe a little foolish.

Despite all this education about STIs, nobody on the planet is happy to get one. The social stigma of STIs remains, and most people still shudder at the very thought of them.

In a way, that's good. I *want* you to shudder. And to have safe sex *every* time. But if you do end up unlucky, remember: It doesn't make you a bad person. Go get treated right away. Your doctor won't judge you. And you deserve to be healthy.

IF YOU'RE BARE DOWN THERE . . . BE AWARE

In chapter 1 we talked about the rage for Brazilian bikini waxes—the removal of most or all of your pubic hair. But the short and curlies may actually provide some small defense against STIs. It's not exactly an electrified barbed-wire fence, but it makes sense that removing the natural barrier can make it easier to contract certain infections, especially those requiring skin-to-skin contact, like HPV and herpes. (Note that there aren't any official scientific studies to support this, so right now it's just a theory.) Plus, microscopic nicks in the skin from shaving or waxing may also increase susceptibility to these infections. I'm not saying don't go Brazilian, but if you do, be even more vigilant in protecting yourself south of the border.

A NOTE FOR GAY TEENS

In this chapter you'll notice I often refer to boyfriends or male partners. I don't mean to exclude lesbians, who make up about 2 to 4 percent of my patients, and the population in general. But since a large majority of my patients are straight, I tend to use the term "boyfriend" since that's the term most of my patients use when we talk.

If you're lesbian or bisexual, please know that it's just as important for you to practice safe sex—and maybe even *more* important, since gay teens are often victims of medical discrimination and are undertreated. (See my note in chapter 9.) Be vigilant about your own health. You deserve it.

CHLAMYDIA: THE STEALTH STI

Can you have a "minor" STI? A lot of teens mistakenly think that since chlamydia isn't visible, doesn't hurt, and is cured easily, it's no big deal. Sort of like getting a bad cold.

Unfortunately, it *is* a big deal *because* it isn't visible and doesn't usually hurt. You don't even suspect you have it. Chlamydia does its dirty work inside your body, potentially scarring and damaging your fallopian tubes. Untreated it can lead to pelvic inflammatory disease (PID), a severe condition that affects the uterus, fallopian tubes, and ovaries, and may lead to infertility. Imagine how you (and your future husband!) will feel down the line when a fertility doctor says there's scarring in your tubes or uterus because of your past sexual choices. If you decide you want a family, you don't want your past sexual behavior coming back to haunt you.

 DID YOU KNOW?
Teens Don't Think Chlamydia Is Serious

A recent study of high schools found that only 19 percent knew that chlamydia can lead to infertility! What *are* they teaching you in "health class" these days? After reading this chapter, I hope you'll test better (in more ways than one . . .).

CHLAMYDIA: TESTING AND TREATMENT

Nobody ever makes an appointment to see me about chlamydia—since it has no obvious symptoms, my patients never even know they have it until they see me. That's why gynecologists routinely test our sexually active patients every six months. It's an easy, fast, painless test: We touch a Q-tip to the opening of the cervix for ten to twenty seconds and then send it for a culture or DNA test. (The throat should also be cultured, since oral sex is a very common and effective way of passing along this infection.) BTW, there's also a special urine test for chlamydia, but the Q-tip culture is more common.

If the test comes back positive, you have chlamydia and need antibiotics. I usually prescribe azithromycin (also known as Zithromax), which can be taken in just one dose. (I favor the single dose route because I know my patients will take a single pill, but I can't always be sure that they'll take antibiotics twice a day for seven days, which they need to do to be fully cured.)

If you're treated for chlamydia, your partner(s) should be, too.

After you take your antibiotics, you need to practice safe sex, or abstain from sex altogether, for a period of four to six weeks. After about three months, I retest my patients to be certain the bacteria are gone. This retesting is really important for teens and not something to blow off. Sometimes if your partner isn't treated or you don't abstain for a while after treatment, the disease can come back and you may need another round of antibiotics.

 DR. ASHTON'S SAFE SEX PLAYLIST

- Oral sex does not equal safe sex.
- Anything you can get from sexual intercourse you can also get from oral sex.

- Many teens believe that oral sex is "not really sex" or is "much safer than real sex." Obviously, this couldn't be further from the truth. See chapter 8 for information on how to have safe oral sex.

AREN'T YOU GLAD I'M NOT YOUR MOTHER?

If I had a teenage daughter diagnosed with chlamydia, I'd call her boyfriend's parents and tell them myself. Yep. Embarrassing and humiliating as it is, I would make sure the family knew. That's because this is an infectious, contagious disease that is reportable to the state health department. That boy needs to be treated before he spreads the disease—no matter how humiliating it is to everyone else involved. I'd feel bad humiliating my daughter, of course. But as I tell my patients: If you're going to behave like an adult and have sex, you need to accept the adult consequences—including awkward and difficult conversations and situations. Even if it means having your mother call your boyfriend's parents about an STI.

DO YOU HAVE TO MAKE A FEDERAL CASE OF IT?

Well, not a federal case. But a state case, yes. In every state, if you test positive for chlamydia, the testing lab will report it to the state health department. The government considers this disease such a threat that it keeps paperwork on who has it and how it was treated. Of course, the state doesn't publish these names. But knowing that the government has a file on your sexual health is enough to make anyone uncomfortable.

FACTS ABOUT CHLAMYDIA

- Might produce no symptoms
- May cause scarring of fallopian tubes
- Can cause future problems with fertility
- Is reported to the state health department
- Is easy to treat with antibiotics

THWART THE WARTS: AVOIDING HPV AND GENITAL WARTS

My patient Mary came to me at the ripe old age of fourteen. She'd told her mother that "her bottom hurt," so her mother brought her in. When I examined her, I wasn't prepared for what I found. This poor girl's genitals were covered (and I mean *covered*) with genital warts. In the medical world we'd describe her genitals as being "carpeted" with warts, because they spread like a rug from her vagina to her rectum. Although Mary was still technically a virgin, she'd gotten naked with her much-older boyfriend on more than one occasion, with this horrifying result.

I prescribed a very strong cream, but after several months there was no improvement and the warts had started to spread into her rectum. I told her that we should consider laser surgery to remove the warts. She kept putting off the appointment. When she finally scheduled the surgery and came for her preoperative visit, I couldn't believe my eyes: The warts had completely vanished! This sometimes happens in young, healthy girls. Mary dodged a major bullet and learned a serious lesson about how problematic genital warts can be.

HPV Is Linked to Cancer

TRUE. HPV causes cervical, throat, and anal cancer, but in a recent study only 27 percent of high school girls knew that.

Genital warts, also known as condyloma, are caused by the human papillomavirus (HPV), which is by far the most common sexually transmitted infection in the United States. HPV is also responsible for abnormal Pap smears and cervical cancer—the second most common cancer found in women worldwide. That's one reason why the HPV vaccine is increasingly being used (see below). A quarter of women ages fourteen to nineteen have had HPV and some 45 percent of women ages twenty to twenty-four have it. About half of sexually active adults will have the infection at some point. Yikes! In other words, it's as common as a cold.

Think that sounds bad? It gets worse. As Mary found out, you don't have to have actual penetrative intercourse (where the penis penetrates the vagina) to get it. Because the HPV virus is passed by direct, skin-to-skin contact, even condoms don't always stop it, for several reasons:

1. Condoms don't cover every skin surface.
2. Many couples don't use condoms until the "last minute" (right before penetration), so the virus can be passed during foreplay.
3. Sometimes you don't even need genital-to-genital contact to get the virus. Occasionally it passes from hands or fingers to the genitalia. So obviously condoms don't help in that case.

All this does NOT mean that condoms are useless: They're the *only* way, besides abstinence, to avoid HPV and other sexually transmitted infections. In this case they provide *some* protection—just not 100 percent protection (just like they don't provide even close to 100 percent protection against pregnancy).

Here's another tricky thing about HPV: Sometimes you won't have visible symptoms. But even if you don't have a visible wart, you can still pass it on. (And even if your partner doesn't have a visible wart, he can give it to you.) No wonder it's so easy to catch. After all, if you noticed your partner had visible warts on or near his penis, you probably wouldn't have sex with him. Likewise, not many guys would have intercourse with a girl who had obvious genital warts.

But most of the time you can't see or feel HPV: It can be asymptomatic, which is a fancy medical way of saying that it might produce no symptoms. Therefore someone can have it and not know it. This is why if your boyfriend promises you he's clean, it might not be a conscious lie. He may not *know* he has HPV. It doesn't mean he's untrustworthy—just naive. Likewise, if you get HPV, it doesn't mean you're promiscuous—just that HPV is *everywhere*. It also may not mean that your boyfriend was cheating on you. You might have picked it up from a previous boyfriend. HPV can lie dormant in your system for years, making it very difficult to figure out who gave it to you.

There are two tiny bits of good news about HPV: One, it probably won't cause any implications later with pregnancy or childbirth. And two, you and your boyfriend probably won't keep passing the infection back and forth like a cold: Your immune systems probably will build up a defense against the strain of the disease you've both picked up (but not against new strains of HPV—and there are more than one hundred types, thirteen of which are associated with cancer).

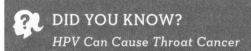

DID YOU KNOW?
HPV Can Cause Throat Cancer

HPV is a common cause of cancer of the vocal cords! In the throat. Guess how it gets there?

It's pretty easy to tell when you have an obvious, external HPV wart. Typically vulvar HPV can include one or more warty-looking growths, ranging in size from a pinhead to a cluster of small warts the size of pencil erasers. Usually flesh-colored, genital warts have a rough, velvety texture, and an irregular border.

Genital warts can be located anywhere in the genital region—at the top of the pubic hair line, in the area around the rectum, or around the inner thighs. In severe cases warts can spread to block the urethra (the urine opening), enter the lower vagina, or even grow into the rectum. These extreme cases can cause pain and bleeding, and they require ongoing medical attention and treatment—sometimes even surgery.

As you can imagine, my patients with genital warts usually want to curl up and die of embarrassment. Mary, for instance, didn't come see me sooner because she didn't want her mother to know. Don't make this mistake. If you have genital warts, put your health first, and deal with your parents or the social issues later. Occasionally, as in Mary's case, the warts go away on their own. But even if this happens, you still need to see a doctor. Your gynecologist will want to know you've had it and be ready to treat it if it comes back.

Luckily, a variety of treatments can help if you contract HPV (plus there's a vaccine—see below). The treatments target the major symptom— the warts—and not the disease itself, for which there's no cure. You just have to wait it out, like waiting to get over a cold.

With Mary we started with medications, which are less aggressive and invasive than surgery. The most common medications prescribed for genital warts include an acid called TCA, a cream called Aldara, or, less often, cryotherapy, which involves freezing the warts. Both the acid and the cream are largely safe and very effective but can take some time before they work. The acids work between 60 and 80 percent of the time, but they need to be applied for several weeks.

Laser surgery, which I recommended for Mary when the medications didn't work, is a more aggressive and invasive treatment, but it works well. About 90 percent of the time laser surgery succeeds in clearing the warts.

DID YOU KNOW?
HPV Is Everywhere

- HPV, the virus that causes genital warts, is the most common STI in the United States.
- Up to 85 percent of fifteen- to twenty-five-year-olds have been exposed.
- HPV causes abnormal Pap smears, cervical cancer, and external genital warts.
- HPV also causes cancer of the vagina and vulva.
- HPV is not always preventable by using condoms.
- HPV can be microscopic or invisible.

HPV VACCINATION: A SHOT FOR CANCER

In 2006 a new vaccine against HPV and cervical cancer hit the market and a media frenzy followed. So chances are good that you've at least *heard* of it. Here's how it works and the pros and cons.

The HPV vaccine is a series of three shots in your arm that helps your body build up immunity against four strains of HPV. (There are more than one hundred types of HPV, but the vaccine protects against the four most aggressive, high-risk types, which are linked with most genital warts and cervical cancer.) The vaccine does not contain the live version of HPV, so the vaccine can't give you the virus. Even though the vaccine has only been available in this country since 2006, it was tested and studied in more than twenty thousand girls in five different countries over five years. By August 2008 more than 20 million doses of the vaccine have been given in the United States. Today about one in four teen girls has at least started, if not finished, the series of three shots against the vaccine.

If you get the vaccine, it definitely *does not mean* that you *cannot* get HPV, since it doesn't protect against many milder strains. But it does mean you'd be very unlikely to get cervical cancer.

To develop the full immune protection against the human papillomavirus, you need to receive all three shots within a twelve-month period. Ideally, you get the second shot two months after the first, and the third shot four months after the second. But you know how teenage life is: Schedules get in the way. That's OK. As long as you get them all in one year, you're good.

The most common side effects include pain and swelling at the injection site and fainting (but we don't know if this is actually from the vaccine or a side effect from jittery nerves about the shot).

VACCINATION PROS

- You probably won't get cervical cancer. (Having the HPV vaccine also helps protect against warts, vaginal cancers, and vulvar cancers.)
- You're less likely to get external genital warts, which are embarrassing and also annoying to treat.
- You're less likely to have abnormal Pap smears, which can lead to extensive cervical surgery.

WHAT'S THE BIG DEAL ABOUT ABNORMAL PAP SMEARS?

The big news about the vaccine is that it can prevent cervical cancer. But it can also prevent the abnormal Pap smears that sometimes occur before cancer appears—and avoiding abnormal Pap smears, and the surgery they sometimes require, is better for your future reproductive health.

Let me explain. Three years after you become sexually active or after you turn twenty-one, your doctor will perform regular Pap smears—a quick, simple, painless test—to make sure the cells of your cervix are normal. If your Pap smears show signs of abnormality, that can be a sign of cervical cancer to come.

Although only four thousand women a year die of cervical cancer, hundreds of thousands of women have abnormal Pap smears every year. Abnormality is rated on a spectrum from low to high. If your Pap smear shows only a low level of abnormality, then your doctor might just wait and repeat the Pap smear in six to twelve months, or he or she might order some tests (including one called colposcopy, where the doctor examines your cervix with a microscope) and regular retests.

But if your Pap smear showed a high level of abnormality, you may require a biopsy or even surgery to remove the abnormal cells from your cervix, because abnormal cells might develop into cancer. For girls under twenty-one new medical standards recommend waiting, and trying to avoid biopsy or surgery unless cancer is present. That's because surgery on your cervix can cause problems with pregnancies later in life. Although the cervix heals well, it can still carry a grudge and make life difficult later, creating trouble with pregnancy or delivery even years after surgery. Unfortunately, because these "wait and see" recommendations are new, many doctors still aren't aware of them and treat teens with abnormal Pap smears like adult women.

Meanwhile, even the new medical guidelines don't account for whether someone has been vaccinated against HPV—which would put them in the lower risk group of cancer and might allow more teens to avoid tests, biopsies, and surgeries.

VACCINATION CONS

In my opinion, the way the vaccine was marketed and advertised as "the cervical cancer vaccine" unfairly played on people's fears of cancer. There are other ways to prevent cervical cancer: Don't ever have sex (OK, not realistic) or always have safe sex (which will at least reduce your chances). People sometimes forget cervical cancer is caused by an STI. I think it's important to remember and do something about the cause.

Second, there have been rare reports of very serious reactions in teens to the vaccine, including paralysis or coma. These have not been fully explained. However, for the girls who believe the vaccine adversely affected them, it's a very big deal. After all, they got the vaccination to avoid a disease and protect their good health.

To date, more than 20 million doses of the vaccine have been given, approximately 600 cases of which have had serious consequences. But it's not clear exactly what caused these consequences or how closely they were linked to the actual vaccine. For example, by 2009, there were twenty-seven deaths reported among girls who had received the vaccine—but some of those were clearly not related to the vaccine. Several were due to automobile accidents and suicide, for instance. So it's hard to know what negative consequences the vaccine actually carries.

Finally—and this isn't exactly a con—but it's not fully known how long the immune protection will last. Currently we know that girls who were vaccinated seven years ago still have evidence of antibodies (which cause immunity) in their blood. But if these levels drop over time, you may require a booster shot down the road.

In the end, you need to evaluate these risks and benefits for yourself. As a doctor, I think the vaccine is safe and that the benefits outweigh any possible risks. That's why I plan to give the vaccine to both my daughter and my son when they're in their late teens. But I support my patients in whatever they decide to do, and I encourage you to make your own decision, after discussing it with your doctor and your parents.

That's what my patient Shani, an orthodox Jew, is working on right now. We talked about the HPV vaccine at her last visit. She thought she wouldn't really need it; at nineteen she was a virgin and she planned to stay one until she got married. No risk. No problem. I told her that made perfect sense from her standpoint. I also pointed out that there's no way to be 100 percent sure her future husband would also be a virgin when they met. Even one sexual partner before her would be enough to give her HPV. And, although no one likes to think this way, the reality of life is that sometimes husbands die or people get divorced. In that case, Shani might re-enter the dating world and could be exposed to HPV later in life. Shani's still thinking about it. I'll support her decision either way.

Meanwhile, I hope you'll approach the HPV vaccination question the same way: Get all the facts, then make your own choice. If you choose not to be vaccinated, you should feel perfectly fine with that decision and not feel guilty about it.

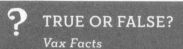

TRUE OR FALSE?
Vax Facts

The HPV vaccine will soon be approved for boys.

TRUE.

The HPV vaccine prevents all strains of HPV and other STIs.

FALSE.

Cervical cancer is the leading cause of cancer death for women in Africa.

TRUE.

Your body makes its own immunity when exposed to HPV.

TRUE. But it's not as high as your immunity will be after the vaccine.

HERPES: YOUR PERMANENT HOUSEGUEST

I'll never forget the day I diagnosed my twenty-year-old patient Samantha with genital herpes. When I gave her the news, she cried so loudly that everyone in the office knew something bad was going on.

"I feel dirty and cheap and ruined," she sobbed, when she could speak again. "Nobody will ever want to be with me again." As her mother held her hand and I wiped away her tears, I told her that getting an infection was not a reflection of her worth.

"It's not something anyone would choose to have," I admitted. "But there are very effective and easy ways to treat this and prevent future outbreaks." It took a lot of time and information, but eventually Samantha made peace with her diagnosis. And so did her next boyfriend, who eventually proposed to her.

Ever had a cold sore? Remember those big, ugly blistery, scabby things near your upper lip or nose, which always pop up at the most embarrassing times? Now imagine the same painful, ugly sore on your privates. That's what herpes is like.

In fact, cold sores and genital herpes are like siblings: They're caused by different strains of the same virus, Herpes Simplex Virus I (HSV-I) and Herpes Simplex Virus II (HSV-II). Although most people think HSV-I causes oral cold sores and HSV-II causes genital herpes, the fact is you can get oral herpes on your genitals and genital herpes on your mouth.

If you're not actually having a herpes outbreak with sores, it's not always easy to confirm whether or not you actually have herpes: Testing for herpes can be difficult, the results are often vague, and the symptoms of genital herpes (aside from the sores) aren't always clear.

One thing that *is* clear: Once you get either strain of the herpes virus, it will stay in your system the rest of your life, and you can expect periodic outbreaks. Sort of like a permanent houseguest who's usually quiet but who suddenly wigs out and smashes all the china now and then. And herpes is an incredibly common houseguest. For instance, about 75 percent of the American population has been exposed to HSV-I. If someone in your immediate family has ever had a cold sore, chances are you've been exposed, too, even if you don't actually break out in blisters. And an incredible one in five Americans has genital herpes.

DID YOU KNOW?
Not Everyone Knows Herpes Is an STI

A recent study of high school girls in South Carolina revealed that almost one out of ten girls did not recognize herpes as an STI![38] Yikes!

 DID YOU KNOW?

A vaccine against herpes is in the works. Stay tuned!

 DR. ASHTON'S HERPES PLAYLIST

I always tell my patients with herpes a few important things:

- It does not make you a bad person.
- It will not prevent you from having a baby later in life.
- Genital herpes is common (unfortunately). One in five Americans has it.
- There is no cure for the herpes virus, but there is good treatment.
- It will not stop someone from loving you, and if it does, you don't want that person anyway!

HERPES SYMPTOMS

My patient Diane, who got herpes at twenty-three, says that when you're having a herpes outbreak, you know it. Her first, she says, felt like "razor blades slicing into my vulva." Ouch. Even before the intense pain, you may feel a general sensation of soreness around your genitals, groin, or pelvis that starts a few days before blisters develop. These blisters are very painful and can be accompanied by burning, itching, swelling, or stinging.

In Diane's case, it hurt when she peed. That's not unusual: In severe cases the opening for the urine, called the urethra, may become so swollen that urination cannot occur. In that event you'd need to be hospitalized with a temporary tube (called a catheter) placed to let the urine out. Patients usually get pain medication and antiviral medication to shorten the length of the outbreak. As with oral cold sores, a typical herpes outbreak lasts about seven days. The blisters take on a greenish or yellowish covering, which eventually crusts over.

? TRUE OR FALSE?

Once you get herpes, you'll always have it.

TRUE. Even if you go years between outbreaks, the herpes virus will always be in your system (this is true for both oral and genital herpes). Most people carrying the herpes virus can expect periodic outbreaks.

You can only transmit herpes when you're having an outbreak.

FALSE. Most people are considered contagious for several days prior to the outbreak and up to two weeks afterward. In fact, new evidence suggests that people may *always* be shedding the virus at low levels and therefore may *always* be contagious.

The Human Pyramid Scheme

Even if you don't have a sore, you could be contagious.

TRUE. People can transmit genital herpes even when they themselves have no symptoms. This process, called asymptomatic viral shedding, is another reason why you *always* need to practice safe sex.

Sometimes herpes produces no symptoms or only vague symptoms.

TRUE.

Herpes can require hospitalization in severe cases.

TRUE.

Antiviral medications can cure herpes.

FALSE. No medication can cure herpes. You'll always have it once you get it. But medications can help prevent or reduce severity of outbreaks.

HERPES: TESTING AND TREATMENT

To diagnose herpes, your doctor will take a good look at the affected area. If blisters are visible, he or she will take a viral culture by scraping off the top of the blister with a Q-tip. If the blister has been there a while, or if the Q-tip didn't scrape off enough material, the culture might come back negative even if you do actually have herpes. Your doctor will also do a blood test for old and new antibodies against both the oral and genital herpes virus.

If your doctor gives you bad news, here's the good news: Herpes can be treated—although not cured—with antiviral medications (the best is called Valtrex) that dramatically reduce or help prevent future outbreaks of either type of herpes. This medication comes in different strengths: a weaker dose to suppress an outbreak and a stronger dose to treat one. There's also a prescription cream called Zovirax, which provides some relief from the painful symptoms of both types of herpes and may shorten outbreaks. Other remedies, such as ice, rubbing alcohol, vitamin E, or lysine supplements have all been used to treat herpes. No tests have proven that they make the sores go away faster, but they might make you feel better.

As my patient Samantha's reaction showed, herpes has emotional effects as well as physical ones. Even though most people know herpes can be acquired nonsexually and that one in five Americans has the disease, the infection still carries a social stigma. But the myths about herpes are wrong: Nice girls can get herpes. Nuns can get herpes. Virgins can get herpes. And you can, too.

I hope someday the social stigma fades. But even if it does, nobody will ever celebrate getting herpes. It's an infection you have for life; there's no cure, only treatment; and it's fairly contagious. As always, prevention is the best medicine. If you always use condoms and keep your number of sexual partners low, your risks of getting this common, embarrassing, and permanent infection will be much lower.

OTHER STIs

There are many, many other STIs: gonorrhea, hepatitis B and C, syphilis, and HIV, to name a few. The only way to prevent any of these is to practice safe sex, using a condom every single time you ever have sex. To lower your odds, be very selective about whom you choose to sleep with. Keep that lifetime number low to reduce your odds of getting any of these.

Here's a little bit more on some STIs you should know about, although I don't see them nearly as often in my office, since they're less common for teens than the Big Three.

HIV/AIDS

Human immunodeficiency virus, or HIV, leads to AIDS (acquired immuno-deficiency syndrome), a disease that has led to the tragic deaths of more than 25 million people around the world since 1981. HIV weakens the body's defenses against serious infections and cancer. This killer is still a leading cause of death in Africa, taking the lives of 1.5 million people, including children, in 2007.[39] There's no cure for HIV, but antiviral drugs have helped drastically decrease death rates in the United States. Still, about 1.1 million people in the United States live with HIV today, according to the Centers for Disease Control—and about 21 percent *don't know they have it*. So someone could infect you without knowing they're infected.

HIV is transmitted by bodily fluids—blood, semen, breast milk, vaginal fluid, and pre-ejaculate fluid. This means that you can get HIV from oral sex, vaginal intercourse, and anal sex. While the virus has been detected in small amounts in tears and saliva, it appears that you cannot get HIV through tears or by kissing. The only way to be sure you won't get HIV (or any STI) is to avoid sex altogether with anyone who carries HIV. If you're thinking about having sex with someone, it's a good idea to ask that person to get tested for HIV and other STIs, and show you the results. (If he's not willing to go get tested, it's a good sign you don't want to be in a relationship with him anyway, let alone have sex with him.)

Short of saying no to sex, condoms are the only way to reduce the chances of getting HIV—or any other STI. Use them every time.

TESTING AND TREATMENT

The HIV test is quick and simple—just a blood test or oral swab. Waiting for those results is the hard part. Unless you're in an emergency situation in a hospital, results normally take a week or two. If you know you've been exposed and your test comes back clean, your doctor might want to test you again in a month, three months, six months, and a year—because sometimes the virus takes that long to appear in the blood.

The American College of Obstetricians and Gynecologists recommends routine testing for women ages nineteen and older, and for teens who are sexually active.

If you do have AIDS, a lifelong course of antiviral medications can keep the disease from progressing into full-blown, often fatal, AIDS.

 QUIZ

Which of these Protect Against STIs?

A. Oral contraceptive pills (aka the pill)
B. The "shot"
C. Always using condoms
D. Using condoms "most of the time"
E. "Pulling out"
F. The cervical cancer vaccine (for all types of HPV and other STIs)

ANSWER: C. Only **using condoms all the time** will protect you effectively against STIs.

GONORRHEA

Like chlamydia, gonorrhea is a sexually transmitted infection so common and worrisome that it's automatically reported to the state department of health, so health officials can track the spread of cases in each state. If you pick it up, the government will have a permanent record of this aspect of your sex life.

If that's not a good enough reason to avoid this bacteria, consider its serious impact on your health. If not detected and treated, gonorrhea can scar the fallopian tubes and cause infertility or sterility. It can also lead to arthritis, meningitis (which affects the brain), and endocarditis (which affects the heart valves). Unfortunately, it can be hard to detect: In 30 to 40 percent of cases it doesn't cause any symptoms.

Gonorrhea is caused by a bacteria, so it can be treated with antibiotics (unlike viruses, like herpes and HIV). Your cervix, anus, and throat are all vulnerable to this bacteria, so don't think that avoiding vaginal sex will help you avoid it (or any other STI). It won't. Depending on where you get it, symptoms can include sore throat, thick, yellow-green vaginal discharge, itching, burning, or irregular vaginal bleeding. You might also feel the need to pee more often than usual.

Typically, gonorrhea symptoms start anywhere from two days to three weeks after you have sex with someone carrying it.

TESTING AND TREATMENT

I check my sexually active patients for gonorrhea every six months as a routine precaution. Since, like chlamydia, you could have it and not know it, such routine tests are crucial. It's a quick, painless test: Just a little Q-tip inserted in the cervix for twenty seconds, or a throat culture just like your pediatrician does for strep. Doctors can also check your urine for gonorrhea, but that's less accurate than a Q-tip culture.

The good news (if there is any) about gonorrhea is that it's easy to treat with a very common antibiotic, such as Cipro (pills) or Rocephin (injected). And 90 to 95 percent of the time these treatments cure the disease. Just to be sure, doctors will usually retest in three to seven days to make sure all the bacteria have been killed. If you get gonorrhea, your sexual partner needs to be retreated as well or he'll just keep reinfecting you. This means one of those awkward conversations: You'll need to tell him that you were diagnosed with gonorrhea and he'll need to see his doctor immediately for treatment.

A FEW OTHER NASTIES
TO KNOW ABOUT

If you think this chapter's been scary, just think—there are many, many other STIs I didn't have room for here. Like syphilis. Once a major health threat, syphilis can now be treated with antibiotics and is far less of a modern concern. But you definitely don't want it—it causes sores and a rash in the early stages, and if undetected it can lead to paralysis, dementia, even death. Then there's hepatitis B and hepatitis C, different viruses that are spread by sex or other activities where your blood might mingle with someone else's (like sharing razors or needles or getting a tattoo). Both can cause flulike symptoms. Sometimes hepatitis B or C goes away quickly, like a cold. But both can become a chronic condition that damages your liver or, in the case of hepatitis C, can even kill you. Other conditions, such as trichomonas, a common STI caused by a parasite, may not be life threatening but can cause annoying symptoms, like foul-smelling discharge, vaginal irritation, and pain during urination.

PUT YOURSELF FIRST:
ALWAYS USE CONDOMS

OK, this might not have been the most fun chapter to read. But I really want you to understand how STIs work, in all their gory detail, so you can protect yourself.

I don't have room here to describe every single thing you can get from sex, but I hope you'll go and learn the facts: Try www.WebMD.com or the government-sponsored Web site on sexually transmitted infections, www.cdc.gov/std.

STIs TO RECOGNIZE

THE THREE MOST COMMON

Chlamydia

Herpes

HPV

OTHER SERIOUS STIs

Gonorrhea

Hepatitis B

Hepatitis C

HIV/AIDS

Syphilis

Trichomonas

Above all, I want you to make sure you always practice safe sex. Always use two forms of birth control—and make one of them condoms. True, condoms aren't 100 percent effective against all STIs. They don't cover every skin surface and sometimes they break or slip. But they're a lot better than nothing—and they're the *only* chance you have to protect yourself from infection and disease once you've decided to have sex. Likewise, you need to know about dental dams (see chapter 8) for oral sex.

Of course, the best way to avoid STIs is to use good judgment and self-control. If you haven't yet become sexually active, wait as long as you can. The longer, the better. (Remember: I'm only saying this for your health. If no one ever got an STI or suffered other serious consequences from sex, I wouldn't care when you start.) If you've already had sex, remember that you don't have to sleep with every guy you have a crush on—that's a great way to wind up with a really unfortunate infection and low self-esteem, too. Be selective. Have high standards.

Finally, if you reach a point in a relationship where you don't want to use condoms (not that I recommend this, but I do live in the real world), ask your boyfriend to get tested for STIs—and ask to see the results in black and white. This is no iron-clad guarantee that he'll stay clean (cases like Shannon's are sadly common). But it does send him the message that your health is your number one priority, and if he really cares about you, your health should be a top priority for him, too. Remember, if you don't take care of yourself, no one else will, either. Only you can protect yourself and your health.

YOUR BODY'S LIFETIME WARRANTY:

Staying Healthy for Life

CHAPTER 11

NO WEIGH

Loving the Body You Have

ne of my patients, Anita, seventeen, has been struggling with her weight for four years.

Medically, her weight is in the normal, healthy range for her height. But her figure could be considered on the fuller side and she desperately wants to lose a few pounds. It doesn't sound like much, but for her it's a very big deal.

Anita takes great care of herself. She bikes, walks, or takes a Pilates class almost every day. And she has terrific eating habits—I don't think she's looked twice at a Snickers bar in years. Still, it's hard for her to lose weight, partly because she has a low-level hormonal disorder.

At our most recent visit, she asked me about those all-protein diets.

"I wouldn't recommend them," I said. "Those diets are usually pretty high in fat and some actually tell you to avoid a lot of fruits and vegetables. Maybe they work in the short term, but they could do long-term damage to your body." Plus, I pointed out, nobody can eat just steak, chicken, and pork forever. "The pounds come back as soon as you start eating normally again."

In the end Anita decided to stay the course and stick with her healthy eating and active lifestyle—even if she keeps her fuller figure. She's not completely at peace with it (and now and then she asks me about other fad diets), but she knows she's doing what's right for her body. And she's slowly learning to love the body she has.

Anita is typical of my teen patients. Each and every one of them worries about her weight in some way. A few really are obese and need to lose thirty or more pounds to avoid health problems. Others are underweight and can't gain even when they try. A few have serious eating disorders. But the vast majority are like Anita—already in their healthy weight zone but struggling to love the body they're in.

Our society doesn't make it easy for teens (or grown women) to love ourselves the way we are. On one hand, the media bombard us with ultra-skinny supermodels and movie stars, telling us we're all *supposed* to look like we just had the stomach flu for six months. On the other hand, restaurants serve entrees that are big enough to feed an entire family, filling plates so enormous that waitresses can barely carry two at a time.

So how do you make sense of all this and start to feel good about your body? It's simpler than you think.

1. Figure out if you're in your healthy weight zone (see the worksheet below).
2. Exercise most days.
3. Follow my "no weigh" rules for healthy eating, below.

Do those three things, and I guarantee you'll start to feel better about your body and yourself. In fact, you really won't even need to step on a scale, except at your regular doctor visits. I call it the "no weigh" solution. I'd even say that most teenage girls don't need scales at all. Instead judge your weight by how you feel and how your (reasonably sized) clothes fit.

So get ready to ditch the scale, put on your workout clothes, and start feeling great.

FASHION MATH, OR, "IF I'M A SIZE ZERO, WHY CAN YOU SEE ME?"

Something strange happened to the laws of mathematics after I left high school. Back then I weighed 118 pounds and wore jeans in size 6. (Note that I'm *not* mentioning my height, so you can't guess what this 118 pounds looked like!) Today I've had two kids (which really changes your body) and I weigh several pounds more. So I wear a bigger size now, right? Nope! I wear a size 2 or 4! According to Fashion Math, I've gone *down* a size!

Somewhere along the line the fashion world decided to tell women they've gotten smaller. Apparently we're supposed to be so giddy about the fact that we fit into a smaller size that we'll buy five pairs of jeans instead of one. And get this: As a result of the new Fashion Math, a lot of people who used to wear a size 2 or 4 actually wear size 0 jeans now. The scientist in me can't get my head around that. In the math world, zero means . . . well, zero. Nothing. It doesn't exist. So tell me—how can a body exist in the world and be a size zero? To me, if I fit into size zero jeans, that would mean I didn't have a body. I'd be invisible. As a mom, this could come in handy (imagine what I could catch my kids doing!), but as a woman, I'd really prefer to exist. Wouldn't you?

HOW MUCH FUEL DO YOU NEED?

To determine if you're a healthy weight, you need to know some basics about energy, calories, muscle, and fat.

Let's start with energy. Bodies are like cars. Some are like hybrids and get a lot of mileage out of just a little gas. Others are like Hummers and take boatloads of fuel to keep them going. Your body's "mileage" is determined by your basal metabolic rate (BMR)—the number of calories you burn at rest, simply by breathing, sitting, and being. (Science review: A calorie is the amount of energy it takes to raise the temperature of one kilogram of water by one degree Celsius at sea level.) Theoretically, if you knew *exactly* how many calories you burn a day (your BMR, plus the calories you burn walking around, exercising, etc.), you'd know precisely how much you could eat without gaining weight. You could eat almost exactly as much as you burned and not gain weight.

The reality of your body's wonderful machinery, however, is much more complicated. Your body actually wants to exist in a "steady state" or stable environment. So it's not easy to gain or lose significant amounts of weight. It's also tough to figure out exactly how much one person can eat, because bodies vary as widely as car models. Your best friend, the Ferrari, might burn more calories just sitting around than do you, the Mini Cooper, simply because she has a different body type and different genes. Athletes typically burn more calories than bookworms of the same height and weight, because athletes have more lean muscle mass, which burns more calories at rest. (See the box on the miracle of weight training, pages 233–234.) The most frustrating part of all this is that some people just have great calorie-burning genes. They can scarf all the potato chips, french fries, and ice cream they want without gaining a pound, while others have to watch every single thing they put in their mouths. When it comes to metabolism, life is so not fair. Still, you *can* learn to care for and love the body you've got. Here's how.

YOUR HEALTHY WEIGHT: BODY MASS INDEX

With more body types than car models out there, it's not always obvious what a healthy weight might be. So doctors look at the ratio of your height and weight, then compare it to other people like you to see if you're in the healthy zone.

This system is called the Body Mass Index. It's an easy calculation where you divide your weight in kilograms by your height in meters squared. (OK, it sounds complicated, but it's easy to do. See the worksheet below. If you don't feel like doing the math, go to www.cdc.gov and search on "BMI for teens" to get an online calculator.)

Typically, the lower your BMI, the less body fat you have. While you need a certain amount of body fat to be healthy, generally speaking you want it to be on the lower side. For adults (people twenty and older), a BMI of 18.5 to 24.9 is normal and healthy. Lower is underweight. Higher is overweight. A BMI over 30 is obese (that is, the person is so overweight that they may have serious health problems).

For teens the calculation isn't quite so straightforward, since teen bodies are still growing and are even more different from each other than adult bodies are. Instead of just looking at your BMI number, your doctor will compare it to the BMI of other people your age to determine what's healthy and normal. If you're below the 85th percentile (that is, if 15 percent or more of all teens your age and height weigh more than you do), you're considered to have a healthy weight. If you're in the top 5 percent, you're obese; if you're in the bottom 5 percent, you're underweight. The CDC site on BMI for teens and children can show you where your normal range is.

HEALTHY BMI RANGE FOR CHILDREN AND TEENS

WEIGHT CATEGORY	PERCENTILE
Underweight	Less than 5th percentile (fewer than 5 percent of teens your age and height weigh less than you do)
Healthy weight	5th to 85th percentile
Overweight	85th to 94th percentile (15 percent or fewer teens your age weigh more than you do)
Obese (so overweight that serious health problems may result)	95th percentile or higher

Source: The Centers for Disease Control

For example, if you're sixteen years old, five feet six inches tall, and weigh 120 pounds, your BMI is 19.4. At the CDC Web site, you'll find that puts you in the 35th percentile for girls your age—healthy!

Once you know your BMI, you may want to check it every year or so to see where you fall compared to last year. This is one area of life where you really want to strive for the middle 85th percentile; being at the 95 percentile for BMI can be just as unhealthy as being at the 5 percentile for BMI.

Your BMI gives you a rough idea of where you stand weightwise, but it's far from perfect. It tells you how you compare to everybody else your age and size, but it doesn't account for things like whether you're athletic or whether you have an unusually high or low BMR. Girls with more muscle may have a falsely high BMI number, since muscle weighs more than fat. In fact, when professional athletes measure their BMI, their results often suggest that they're obese, which couldn't be less true!

The healthy range is incredibly wide. My patient Anita (who's seventeen, measures five feet four, and weighs 140) is in the healthy range—but that range goes from 101 to 146 pounds! So BMI is just one piece of the puzzle helping you figure out your best weight. Since Anita has a hormonal imbalance, I'd expect her to be on the high end of the normal range. But I also know she exercises nearly every day and has a very healthy diet. So landing somewhere in the middle makes sense for her. It's also important to take into account elements like genetics and her metabolic rate.

When you factor in all these different variables, plus genetics and personal metabolic rate, it makes sense that there's a wide range of healthy.

DO YOU NEED TO LOSE WEIGHT?

But what if you're *not* healthy? If you're obese or overweight, you need to work with a doctor and a nutritionist to get down to a healthy weight. You'll probably want to develop careful eating habits and start an exercise program. But most of all, you'll want to find someone or something that can help you to get started, stick with it, and stay motivated! The name of the game here is lifelong health and well-being—*not* a number on a scale or a certain size of jeans.

If you're truly overweight or obese, you should also recognize that even small reductions in your BMI can translate into *big* improvements in your overall health. So your journey is just as important as your starting and finishing point. The goal is to move closer to a healthy weight range, not just achieve a target weight.

If you're at the high end of your healthy range, ask yourself if your eating habits are healthy and if you're exercising for thirty to sixty minutes or more most days of the week. If not, do both of those things and see if you lose weight. But if you *are* already eating healthy and exercising most days, it may be time to make peace with your body.

TIPPING THE SCALE: IF YOU'RE OVERWEIGHT

Being at the high end of your normal, healthy range doesn't mean you need to lose weight. But if you fall into the "overweight" or "obese" category, you need to change the way you eat and exercise to get into the healthy range. Lots and lots of medical studies have shown that obesity leads to all kinds of health problems. Physically, the body has to work harder just to live. Over many years this can lead to problems with your heart and blood vessels, including high blood pressure and heart disease. With much more body tissue to nourish, your pancreas has to work harder to produce insulin to process your food and turn it into energy. Meanwhile, the insulin you do have becomes less effective. Together these two processes lead to diabetes, which can lead to kidney and eye problems, heart attack, and stroke.

But wait, that's not all! If you're obese, you may have problems breathing and sleeping and issues with your skin and joints. And you're more likely to have irregular periods and early puberty (a risk factor for breast cancer).

On top of all that—maybe even more important, from a teen's point of view—it's just not fun to feel uncomfortable with your body. Especially in high school.

Unfortunately, it's not easy to lose weight if you're truly obese, because a stubborn combination of genetics, behavior, and environment work against you. When diet and exercise just don't work, I sometimes advise my obese patients to consider Lap-Band surgery, where a band is surgically placed around the upper stomach. While Lap-Band surgery isn't usually offered to teens under the age of eighteen and isn't the answer for everyone, it can be life-saving for many who struggle with true morbid obesity (a dangerous degree of obesity that can cause physical disability and a severely impaired quality of life). Usually morbid obesity means you have a BMI of 40 or more, or that you're one hundred pounds or more over your healthy body weight.

One of my favorite patients, Amanda, was more than one hundred pounds over her ideal healthy weight by the age of fifteen. She'd tried every possible diet known to womankind. Nothing worked. As a result of her weight, Amanda had knee problems, skin problems, menstrual irregularities, and sleep apnea. By the time she was nineteen, she was five feet two inches and weighed 265 pounds. I met with Amanda and her mother and suggested she consider Lap-Band surgery, which many doctors now consider the best treatment for morbid obesity.

I explained that Lap-Band surgery is quick, safe, and easy, and patients usually go home the same day or the day after the operation. The band is adjustable and the entire procedure is reversible. After meeting with a surgeon, a pediatrician, and me, Amanda and her mom decided that surgery was a good option. When I saw her seven months after her surgery, Amanda had lost seventy-three pounds! Her sleep apnea problems had disappeared and her knee pain was lessening. She felt great physically and emotionally and was proud of herself for taking a big step toward better health.

WEIGHTY PROBLEMS: THE RISKS OF OBESITY WHEN YOU'RE A TEEN

Early puberty
Early first period
Irregular periods
Low self-esteem
Low participation in sports and exercise

LATER IN LIFE:
High blood pressure
Heart disease
Diabetes
Stroke
Some cancers

SLIM CHANCES: THE RISKS OF BEING TOO THIN

My patient Cindy had always been a star student, but when she turned thirteen, the stress of adolescence became too much for her. Her parents were splitting up, and Cindy's mother was struggling with self-esteem issues. She constantly criticized both herself and Cindy for not looking their best. Meanwhile, Cindy was losing interest in her classes and getting in trouble at school for the first time. She felt she had no control over her life.

Cindy decided to take control by drastically restricting the amount of food she ate. From a healthy five feet four and 115 pounds, she dropped to 110, then 100, then 96 pounds. At fourteen her periods stopped. Six months later she had a seizure in history class, caused by a severe imbalance in her blood chemistry. Her doctors realized she had anorexia. She was admitted to the hospital for treatment. I started treating her a few years later, after her anorexia was largely under control and her body weight normal, thanks to lots of psychotherapy and hard work on her part. But she'll probably struggle with her eating disorder for the rest of her life.

No one knows exactly what causes anorexia nervosa, bulimia, or other eating disorders. Genetics, stress, and social and psychological factors may all play a role. Still, lots of girls endure the divorce of their parents, struggles at school, and other forms of stress but never develop eating disorders.

What we *do* know is that teens with anorexia have a distorted body image. No matter how much weight they lose, they still see themselves as fat and disgusting. True, many teenagers feel frustrated and anxious about how they look sometimes, but girls with anorexia loathe their looks *all the time*. They literally want to make themselves disappear.

In severe anorexia the body starts to shut itself down. Periods stop or come irregularly, the body stops controlling its temperature well, and mental focus and concentration start to slip. In the worst cases girls with anorexia starve to death. In fact, anorexia has one of the highest death rates of all psychological disorders: As many as 15 percent of people with anorexia die from conditions related to the disease (including suicide).[40]

Bulimia, another common eating disorder where girls go on eating binges then purge their food by vomiting or taking laxatives, shares some symptoms with anorexia. One thing they don't share is significant weight loss: Bulimics often maintain a normal weight. Still, the body fails to get the nutrients it needs and may shut down certain functions.

SYMPTOMS OF EATING DISORDERS

One of the key signs of anorexia is a 15 to 20 percent drop in weight. So if your 120-pound friend drops below 102 or so, you should be worried.

Another sign is bizarre dressing. Girls with anorexia will often wear big, heavy, loose clothing even on hot days. Giant sweatshirts hide their wasted figures and provide much-needed warmth for their bodies. At critically low body weight, the part of the brain in charge of regulating body temperature starts to shut down. People with eating disorders are always cold.

Girls with bulimia may not show much weight loss, since the binge-and-purge cycle may keep them at a stable weight. A girl with bulimia may make frequent trips to the bathroom or leave the table immediately after eating. She might have scrapes on her knuckles from sticking her finger down her throat to induce vomiting. Her breath may smell fruity or just plain bad. In severe cases she may have dental problems: Stomach acid, brought up by vomiting, is very bad for teeth. In rare cases blood chemistry changes can also lead to serious heart problems or even a stomach rupture from vomiting.

SIGNS OF EATING DISORDERS

If you think you or a friend may have anorexia or another eating disorder, please tell an adult whom you trust about your concerns. It may turn out to be nothing. But eating disorders can be life-threatening, so better safe than sorry. Look out for the symptoms below.

- Body weight drops 15 to 20 percent or more below normal
- Wearing heavy loose-fitting clothing
- Excessive exercising
- Rigid eating habits
- Obsession with calories
- Sleeping a lot
- Bad breath
- Irregular or stopped periods
- Anemia
- Poor hair or nail quality
- Stomach or joint pain
- Headaches
- Difficulty concentrating

THE ATHLETIC TRIAD

One of my patients, JoJo, is a competitive swimmer for a Division I college. She practices two or three hours every day. When she came to me for her first visit, she was only having three or four periods a year. After doing some tests, we determined that JoJo was showing the "athletic triad." This situation affects girls who exercise a lot, have relatively low body weight, and stop menstruating. Basically these girls aren't getting enough calories to stay healthy because they're exercising so much. Consciously or sub-consciously, they're putting athletics ahead of their overall health. They burn many more calories than they take in, with potentially very serious effects on their overall health. Their bodies don't produce normal levels of estrogen, putting them at risk for weak bones and fractures. Their blood chemistry can become abnormal (as it can in anorexics or bulimics), which can lead to heart problems, seizures, or death.

JoJo was concerned about gaining any weight. She believed that even one extra pound could slow her down in the pool. But her irregular periods showed her body wasn't getting the estrogen it needed to build strong bones, which could lead to osteoporosis later in life (see chapter 6). I recommended that she start a low-dose hormone pill to create regular periods and help protect her bones. JoJo was afraid the hormones would make her put on pounds, but I assured her that most forms of the pill don't cause weight gain—and indeed, we found a formulation where she didn't gain weight.

Giving her a "pill period" and possibly helping her bones was the easy part, but it didn't address the diet and exercise imbalance. *That* was the harder part. JoJo worked with a nutritionist to modify her eating habits and eventually worked out a balance where her body got the fuel it needed to stay healthy. Along the way she learned that more isn't always better—and that too much of anything (even swimming) can be potentially harmful.

SHADES OF GRAY

Most people have heard of anorexia or bulimia, but very few realize that eating disorders aren't always black and white. They're not like pregnancy—where you either *are* pregnant or you're not. Instead there's a range of attitudes about eating. It's possible to have a very unhealthy attitude about food (for instance, spending all your time preoccupied with food, obsessively counting calories or exercising, or engaging in certain food rituals) without developing a life-threatening eating disorder. But just because you don't have a clinical disorder doesn't mean you're happy. I don't want you to waste your incredibly valuable energy and time focused on food when that same energy could go to your studies, your friends, your family, or the novel you dream about writing. My goal for my patients, and for you, isn't simply to *not* have an eating disorder. I want you to have a healthy attitude toward food that will get you in great shape and help you feel your best about yourself. Here's how.

NO WEIGH: DR. ASHTON'S FIVE SIMPLE RULES FOR HEALTHY EATING

News flash: Eating healthy isn't complicated. You don't have to follow some fad diet to the letter. You don't have to count every calorie or become an amateur nutritionist. You don't even have to suffer. You just need to follow a few very simple rules. Do it and I guarantee you'll feel better about yourself. And you'll find it much easier to stick to your healthy weight. I promise.

 DR. ASHTON'S FIVE HEALTHY EATING RULES

Most diets say "Don't, don't, don't!" Instead try these five dos for a lifetime of healthy weight. I'll tell you more about each of these tips below, but here's a quick cheat sheet.

1. Find an exercise you love and do it most days.
2. Eat from the farm, not the factory. Choose foods that look like something that came from a tree, a field, or a barn instead of packaged, processed food. Pick fresh fruits over fruit bars, raw veggies over veggie chips, water over soda, etc.
3. Eat a rainbow of foods. Incorporate as many different colors of food as you can, every day. (We're talking natural colors—red, green, and blue M&M's don't count!)
4. Drink six to eight glasses of water every day.
5. Eat smart portions. A serving size should be approximately the amount of food you can hold in your cupped hands. Eat roughly that much per meal.

Rule One: Find an Exercise You Love

The first and most important rule about healthy eating isn't about food at all. It's this: Find a physical activity that you like enough to do almost every day. Maybe that's a team sport like soccer or volleyball, maybe it's dancing, horseback riding, Rollerblading, jogging, or—my favorite!—karate. Exercise has such an important effect on your body that in some ways it's even *more* important than what you eat.

In the old days they used to say "you are what you eat." But today we're finding more and more that "you are what you *do*." If you sit around all day like a sack of potatoes, guess what? Your body will *look* like a sack of potatoes. On the other hand, if you run or swim or bike or lift weights, you'll start to look more and more like a runner or swimmer or biker or other athlete. You'll be stronger, fitter, and—bonus!—you'll be able to eat more without gaining weight.

Regular exercise brings so many other benefits that it really does look like a miracle cure. Studies have shown that girls who participate in sports are much less likely to smoke, drink, or use drugs. If you're athletic, you're more likely to have higher self-esteem and less likely to have sex at an early age. And if you exercise regularly, you may do better in school: One study showed that high school students who worked out vigorously before class showed more improvement than students who didn't.[41] Not to mention that daily exercise probably will make you happier: Many studies have shown that exercise works as a natural antidepressant.

LIFTING WEIGHTS LETS YOU EAT MORE

How would you like to burn more calories while just sitting still? Sound too good to be true? Guess again. You *can* up your BMR (basal metabolism rate) through exercise—particularly through weight lifting. Lean muscle mass burns a few more calories when resting than does fat, and day after day those extra calories add up. In the end lifting weights to build your muscles can help you stay in shape even when you're just sitting around watching TV.

Even if weights didn't boost your metabolism, they definitely make a difference in how you look. A fourteen-year-old who weighs 140 pounds and wears a size 8 but who lifts weights and swims competitively has a body that's very different from that of someone the same age and size who knits sweaters for a workout. I guarantee the weight-lifting swimmer will look slimmer and more fit—and be able to eat a lot more without gaining weight!— than the knitter.

SELF-ESTEEM THROUGH SELF-DEFENSE

If you're already in high school, you might feel like it's too late to try a new sport. Or maybe you're just not the team-sports type. Have I got an idea for you: martial arts.

No kidding. That's what I did. I've always admired my pal (and dentist) Patti, not just because she's a fabulous person and lots of fun, but because she has one of the most impressively toned and fit bods I've ever seen. Even her muscles have muscles. She gives all the credit to karate and weight lifting, both of which she's done for years. After hearing her rave about karate, I had to try it, too (some types of peer pressure never go away). Now I'm a convert. I love that I don't have to squeeze into skimpy exercise clothes. Plus, I get to progress at my own pace, without any pressure to keep up with a team. And I love having a goal to work toward. (Now I've reached a high degree blue belt and Patti's almost a black belt!) Not to mention that learning self-defense basics is a great idea for any girl or woman. What's not to like?

How Much Is Enough—or Too Much? Most current recommendations urge you to work out almost every day, for up to an hour and to do a combination of weight lifting and aerobic exercise (running, biking, swimming, or any other exercise that gets your heart pumping). That's great, but if you can't do it, just do *something*. Walk briskly a few nights a week with your mom or a girlfriend. Bike to school and back a few days a week. Jog a mile after school. Just do something.

In addition to karate (see the box on the facing page), I think running and jogging are great exercise for teens. Running doesn't cost anything (except running shoes, which, I admit, can add up). Plus, you can do it with friends. Talking while running makes the workout that much more challenging—a good thing! You don't have to run a marathon to get in shape (although that's a great goal if you're so inclined). Just jogging a couple of miles several times a week will get you into good shape. And it's a great way to clear your mind.

If you hate running, here's my advice: Don't run. Find something else you like to do. Nobody can stick with an exercise regime they hate. These days there are a million exercise options for girls, so I know you can find something you like. I have patients who swim, play soccer, or ride horses, and they're all in great shape. My daughter, Chloë, plays ice hockey and absolutely loves it. So don't think of exercise as a chore or something you dread. Find something you enjoy. If you like doing something, chances are you'll keep doing it and that you'll get good at it. Sticking with things you're good at boosts your mental and emotional health, too.

Another tip: Listen to your body. If you're injured, if something hurts, or if you stop getting your period, your body may be telling you to slow down. And if your grades or family life start to suffer because of the time you spend doing sports, it may be time to reevaluate your priorities. Try to do something every day—but keep it in balance.

Rule Two: Eat from the Farm, Not the Factory (Or, Where Do Twinkies Grow?)

Here's my easy eating tip: Eat only things that are suitable for putting into your body. Chips, soda pop, candy, fried foods—even fruit juices to some extent—all spend most of their lives in a factory, not on a farm. If a food can sit on a shelf for weeks (or months or years!), chances are it has a lot of chemicals and preservatives in it—not stuff you want to put in your body. In general, the closer a food is to something you can recognize (raw or lightly cooked vegetables and fruits, lean meats, milk, yogurt), the better it is for your body. (Twinkies, you'll notice, have almost no resemblance to anything that grows on a tree.)

It's OK to eat processed junk food once in a while. By itself that Krispy Kreme donut isn't so horrible if your typical lunch is fresh fruit and a turkey sandwich (hold the mayo!). But it's not a great side dish to a daily menu of french fries and nachos. So as a general rule, on a day-to-day basis, try to not even look at chips, soda pop, sugary fruit juices, candy, fried food, packaged cookies, and stuff like that. They do nothing good for your body. It's like putting the wrong kind of fuel in your car: It'll run for a while, but eventually everything breaks down.

Rule Three: Eat a Rainbow

A simple way to find healthy foods is to include a wide range of colors in your diet. Green from veggies like broccoli, peas, and spinach; red from strawberries, beets, red peppers, and pomegranates; yellow for squash, yellow peppers, pineapple, and mangos. Blueberries, blackberries, red chard, purple cabbage. You get the picture—in living color. Nutritionists recommend you have several different hues on your plate at any given meal.

That's because foods with various colors contain a wide variety of nutrients that you could never get by eating just one color. What you especially want to avoid is a "white" diet (followed by some in my own family), made up mostly of pasta, white bread, potatoes, mayonnaise, and so on. Most of these are starchy foods with lots of empty calories. If most of your foods are white, you're missing out on some major nutrients.

Rule Four: Water, Water, Everywhere

Drink water or sparkling water, not soda. Soda comes from a factory and it's filled with chemicals, sugar, and who knows what. Plus, sodas and sugary juices are a big waste of calories. Even a healthy juice with no sugar or preservatives added may have 100 or more calories. I myself would much rather eat those calories than drink them.

Water, on the other hand, is good for your skin and it can help prevent headaches and help your kidneys do a better job filtering bad stuff out of your blood. Plus, if you drink six to eight glasses of water every day, you'll be less hungry and less likely to fill your tummy with junk.

Do other liquids offer the same benefits? Yes and no. Sodas and high-sugar juices might hydrate you and move food along its path in your intestines—but all that sugar could also be a source of weight gain and fluctuating energy levels. Water is best.

ARE YOU GETTING ENOUGH WATER?

A good way to tell if you're getting enough water is to look at the color of your pee. The darker yellow it is, the more dehydrated you are.

On the other hand, you should know that technically it *is* possible to drink too much water—you can actually die from chugging many gallons of it. Every now and then you'll read about some frat party gone wrong, where pledges are forced to chug gallons of supposedly harmless water and someone dies. This is just one more reason to pursue moderation in all things—even things that *seem* perfectly healthy.

Rule Five: Eat Smart Portions, or "Who Ordered the Truckload of French Fries?"

How often do you eat something? Probably every three to four hours, right? So why do restaurants act like you haven't eaten in a month? When my family of four orders at a restaurant, the plates are so loaded that the waitress usually has to make two trips. Over the past few decades, the American idea of a portion size has ballooned. Back in 1960 the average Coke was 6.5 ounces. Now it's hard to find anything smaller than 20 ounces in a vending machine! Fifty years ago a typical bagel was 2 to 3 ounces: Now it's twice that size.[42]

Meals and portion sizes are just way too big now. But it's easy to fix. Just remember this: The correct portion size for a meal is roughly equal to the amount of food that could fit in your hands when you cup them together in the shape of a bowl. That's your *whole meal*, mind you. Not a double handful of potatoes, a double handful of chicken, and a double handful of stuffing—which is pretty much what you'd be served if you ordered a chicken dinner at any chain restaurant in America these days. That's as many calories as your body needs for almost an entire day. You should think of most restaurant meals as enough for dinner tonight *and* for lunch tomorrow (if not breakfast and dinner, too!).

So forget what your mother told you (just this once!)—don't clean your plate if you're not hungry. Eat until you're satisfied (*not* stuffed—just not hungry anymore), and then stop.

EAT TO LIVE, DON'T LIVE TO EAT

Ben Franklin's words are more true today than ever. It's all too easy to get into the habit of eating (or drinking) for reasons besides hunger and thirst. Sure, we've all heard of "comfort foods." Lots of people turn to munchies every time they're bored, tired, anxious, worried, nervous, or angry. But eating to make yourself feel better just isn't healthy.

I'm sure you've seen moms try to quiet a screaming toddler with a lollipop or sippy cup. It works pretty well. But if this pattern of appeasing tears with food or sweets continues into later childhood, it can lead to potentially unhealthy patterns. What works for a toddler isn't necessarily healthy for a teenager.

Movies and TV shows don't help us establish good coping mechanisms either. How many times have you seen the broken-hearted girl reach for a pint of chocolate ice cream to soothe her spirits?

Sure, everybody splurges now and then on not-so-nutritious foods. But if you reach for the chocolate or the chips every time you run into a disappointment, tragedy, fight, or stressful event, that's a recipe for bad health. Instead take a walk, call a friend, pick up a hobby, or soothe yourself in other ways. If you find you're always using food as a reward or a soother, consider speaking to a counselor or therapist. Professionals can suggest different coping techniques that don't involve eating.

LOVING THE BODY YOU HAVE

If you were an alien scientist on a research trip to earth, here's what you'd conclude about American women:

- Based on changes in clothing labels, American women are getting smaller.
- Based on restaurant portion sizes, Americans need a lot more food than they used to.
- Based on magazines, movies, and TV, all women are tall and thin and have perfect skin.
- Based on Barbie dolls, American women have a thirty-nine-inch bust, an eighteen-inch waist, and thirty-three-inch hips.[43]
- Based on Bratz dolls, they have big puffy lips (like somebody punched them in the face) and hair grown past their butts.

Fortunately, I'm not an alien scientist. I'm an actual real live human scientist who happens to see a whole lot of bodies of every shape and size. And I'm pleased to report that none of the above is true.

What *is* true is that you don't have to look like a model, an actress, a Barbie, or a Bratz to be beautiful, have friends and a boyfriend, and feel good about yourself. What you do need to do is value yourself enough to eat right, find exercise you enjoy, and take care of your body with all the love and kindness you deserve.

CHAPTER 12

JUST SAY KNOW

Facts on Smoking, Drinking, Drugs, and More

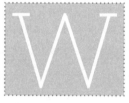hen I was in high school (which wasn't *that* long ago . . .), smokers were everywhere: restaurants, movie theaters, airplanes. I even remember visiting the hospital with my dad and seeing patients smoking. "Huh?" I thought. "Isn't smoking what puts you *in* the hospital?"

That was then, this is now. Chances are you've never even seen an ashtray in a restaurant, since so many states now ban smoking in public places.

Still, plenty of people risk their lives every single day by starting and continuing to smoke. They've got to know it's bad for them: You'd have to be living under a rock to miss the fact that smoking causes cancer, not to mention all kinds of other health problems. Yet more than a million teenagers take up smoking every year.

I don't want you to be one of them. Trust me, it's a million times easier never to start smoking than it is to quit. That's also true of other temptations you may face in high school, like drinking and drugs. Passing these up in the face of peer pressure is a lot easier if you know the facts—not just that they're bad for you but *why* they're bad and how they affect your body from a medical point of view. As I always tell my patients, just say *know*: Learn the facts, decide what's right for your body, and make a plan to stay healthy and safe.

SMOKE AND MIRRORS

Hey! Want to take up a hobby that's really expensive, gives you bad breath, stains your teeth, gives you wrinkles around your mouth, and—oh yeah—can give you lung cancer and heart disease?

Four thousand teens said yes to that question today. Another four thousand will say yes tomorrow. That's how many people aged twelve to seventeen start smoking every day,[44] despite the fact that it causes cancer, shortens your life, and is illegal if you're under the age of eighteen. Many of these young smokers are launching a lifelong bad habit. A study by the Centers for Disease Control showed that 80 percent of smokers start before the age of eighteen.

Here's a quick tour of exactly what happens to your body when you smoke.

The "cancer stick," as my patient Julia calls it, couldn't be simpler: paper wrapped around tobacco, with a filter on the end. Tobacco meets flame, filter meets lips, and smoke floods into the mouth, throat, and lungs.

But the effect of smoke on the body is far from simple—and it's very powerful. From the very first puff of your first cigarette, you start to damage cells and tissues in the mouth, throat, and lungs. First, the smoke paralyzes the cilia in the windpipe—tiny, hairlike structures that sweep back and forth like seaweed and keep dirt, molecules, and mucus from slipping down into the lungs. When cilia meet smoke, they stop working, so all that crud falls down into your lungs. This is why heavy smokers have that wet, gravelly cough. Yuck.

Once the smoke reaches your lungs, you're really in trouble. Tobacco smoke lets off more than fifty cancer-causing substances and thousands of toxic chemicals, including carbon monoxide, which increases your chance of cardiovascular diseases. Not only do these chemicals hurt the lungs themselves, increasing a smoker's risk of lung cancer, emphysema, and other breathing problems,[45] but they also get absorbed by the bloodstream and body tissue. Carbon monoxide, for instance, latches on to blood molecules and deprives the brain of oxygen. And that's just one of the thousands of toxins you're setting loose in your body. Bottom line: Every single cell that comes into contact with nicotine has a chance of becoming cancerous.

So that's what smoking does to the inside of your body. And outside? It doesn't take long for tobacco to start damaging your looks—your teeth turn yellow, you get stains on your lips and fingers, and you start getting wrinkles around your mouth. Not to mention very nasty breath. Frankly, I'm pretty sure these immediate visual effects discourage my patients from smoking even more than the cancer risk.

ARSENIC, CYANIDE, AND BENZENE, OH MY! THE DANGERS OF SECONDHAND SMOKE[46]

It's not just your own health you hurt when you smoke. The surgeon general's office reports that secondhand smoke—given off by the burning end of a cigarette or exhaled by smokers—can cause cancer, asthma, and other serious health problems. Being around secondhand smoke for even a little while—like at a party or a restaurant—can damage blood vessels and increase the risk of heart attack. Just like smoke inhaled by smokers, secondhand smoke includes hundreds of toxic or carcinogenic substances. You don't have to be a scientist to figure out that breathing stuff called formaldehyde, arsenic ammonia, hydrogen cyanide, and benzene can't be good for you. Secondhand smoke kills about 50,000 adult nonsmokers a year, from heart disease and lung cancer, and causes between 150,000 and 300,000 respiratory infections in infants and toddlers. Hundreds of cases of sudden infant death syndrome (SIDS) have been linked to smoking.

DID YOU KNOW?
Smoking Causes at Least Ten Types of Cancer

Everybody knows smoking causes lung cancer. But did you know it also causes many other forms of cancer, too, including cancers of the mouth, throat, voice box, esophagus, pancreas, kidney, bladder, stomach, and cervix, and even a type of leukemia (cancer of the blood)?[47] That's because the cancer-causing chemicals in smoke enter your blood and get transported throughout your entire body.

SMOKING: SHORT-TERM EFFECTS

- Poor lung function
- Poor lung growth
- Increased risk of respiratory infections, coughing, and wheezing
- Faster heart rate at rest
- Stains on teeth, lips, fingers
- Wrinkles
- Bad breath

SMOKING: LONG-TERM EFFECTS

- Lung problems such as bronchitis, emphysema, and lung cancer
- Weaker bones
- Cancers of the throat, mouth, bladder, kidney, esophagus, colon, and cervix (and lungs, of course)
- Menstrual problems
- Earlier menopause

TEEN SMOKING: UP IN SMOKE?

Good news. Teen smoking rates have dropped a lot in the past decade. Today about 22 percent of high school students smoke, down from 36.4 percent in 1997.[48]

SMOKE SIGNALS: WHAT YOUR CIGARETTE SAYS ABOUT YOU

About a million years ago—like, in the 60s and 70s—smoking was supposed to make you seem cool, sophisticated, and worldly. That image is total history. In movies and TV shows today it's almost always the bad guy that smokes, not the hero. Today smoking doesn't say "I'm cool." Instead it gives off three clear messages to your friends . . . probably not the ones you want to send.

1. **"I don't care about my health."** Unless you've been living under that rock, you know smoking is bad for you. Everybody else

knows that, too. And *they* know *you* know. So when people see you smoking, you're telling them "I don't care about my body." And if you don't care, why should anybody else?

2. **"I'm looking for trouble."** It's unusual for a teen smoker to be a straight-A student athlete. I'm not saying it can't happen, but it's the exception, not the rule. Smoking often goes hand in hand with other unhealthy behavior, including alcohol and drug use, higher rates of sexual activity (which lead to higher rates of STIs and pregnancy), and bad grades. In one study teens who smoked cigarettes in the previous month were three times more likely to use alcohol, eight times more likely to smoke pot, and twenty-two times more likely to use cocaine than teens who didn't smoke.[49] With every cigarette you send up signals that you're looking for trouble. It's only a matter of time before it finds you.

3. **"I'm insecure!"** If you're smoking to seem cool or sophisticated, you're actually sending the opposite message. Smoking tells people that you're insecure on some level. It says you're willing to do anything—even something unhealthy—to fit in or seem cool.

Sure, we all feel insecure sometimes. I myself fell victim to more than one unfortunate fashion trend to fit in with my high school friends. Lucky for me, red suede ankle boots don't cause cancer. If you're insecure enough to risk your health just to make a statement or get attention, what else might you end up doing? Don't go down this road—either with smoking or with fashion!

 DID YOU KNOW?

MOST GIRLS WHO SMOKE:
Smoke to feel "cool" and mature
Have parents or relatives who also smoke
Don't plan to graduate from college
Smoke to cope with stress

DID YOU KNOW?
Smoking Can Make You Fat

"I want to quit, but I don't want to put on weight," my patient Shana told me. I hear that a lot. But a recent study found that girls who smoked as teens were more than twice as likely to become overweight later in life than nonsmokers. So smoking may actually hurt, not help, your chances of staying at a healthy weight for life.[50]

DR. ASHTON'S CANCER-STICK PLAYLIST

- Smoking tells your friends that you're insecure and don't care about your body. These aren't just negative messages—they're dangerous ones.
- Smoking makes you ugly: It gives you wrinkles, stains your teeth, and makes your breath stink.
- Smoking a pack a day costs $2,000 a year. Think of all the shoes that could buy you.

QUITTERS ALWAYS WIN

My patient Lynn tried her first cigarette when she was fourteen. She thought she'd be able to keep it to the occasional puff, but pretty soon she was smoking three or four packs a week. She made friends with other smokers her age—friends who were a little older and wilder.

At sixteen Lynn got a crush on Evan, who didn't smoke—and said he'd never date a smoker. She made up her mind to quit.

Her first try lasted about forty-eight hours. "I'd be fine, but then I'd start getting really anxious and feeling like only a cigarette would calm me down," she said. After two days, she told herself, "Just one won't hurt." By the end of the week she was smoking as much as before.

But she wasn't down yet. She read up on how to quit smoking on Web sites like smokefree.gov. Next time she made a plan.

1. She picked a date to stop smoking.
2. She made up an excuse to tell her smoker friends. Yes, in theory she shouldn't have to lie. But then again, in theory, her "friends" shouldn't be pressuring her to smoke. "I told them my doctor said I had asthma, and I had to quit," she confesses. Sometimes a white lie makes life a little easier.
3. She made lots of social plans with friends who didn't smoke.
4. She bought loads of chewing gum, baby carrots, and other crunchy stuff to keep her mouth busy.
5. She took up jogging. "You can't smoke and jog," she told me. If she desperately wanted a smoke, she put on her running shoes instead for a quick run, even if it was just around the block.

This time Lynn's plan worked. She quit. The funny thing was, she never did end up dating Evan. While she was busy hanging out with her nonsmoking friends, she met somebody she liked even more.

"NO THANKS, I REALLY HATE CANCER"

Resist the pressure to start smoking—or aid your efforts to quit—by having a few quick one-liners ready if friends pressure you.

1. "I care about my health and I'm not going to smoke."
2. "I don't need cigarettes to feel cool."
3. "Smoking causes wrinkles and I like to look good."
4. "If you smoke as a teen, you're twice as likely to be overweight as an adult."
5. "I have asthma."

6. "My doctor told me my cough was a complication from smoking."

7. "My parents told me that they wouldn't pay for college if I continued to smoke."

 DID YOU KNOW?

On average, smokers die thirteen to fourteen years earlier than nonsmokers.[51]

IF YOUR PARENTS SMOKE

If your parents smoke, try anything and everything to get them to quit. You may save their lives. Back in college my future husband told his dad he wouldn't come home to visit unless his dad quit smoking. It worked—his dad quit! Tell your parents how much you love them—and that you don't want to lose them early. To make it easier, adults can call in some help that teens don't have—some prescription medications, not approved for teens, can ease withdrawal symptoms (as can nicotine patches or nicotine gum). So talk to your parents about how much you want them to quit. It just might work.

? TRUE OR FALSE?
Smoking

Low-tar cigarettes reduce the risk for lung cancer.

FALSE.

Smoking increases the risk of bone fractures, dental problems, eye problems, and sexual problems.

TRUE.

Smokers live just as long as everyone else.

FALSE. On average, they die thirteen to fourteen years earlier.

White teenage girls are more likely to smoke than black or Latino teenage girls.

TRUE. In one survey, about 22.5 percent of white teenage girls smoked regularly, compared with just 8.4 percent of black teen girls and 14.6 percent of Latino teen girls.[52]

GOING TO POT: THE RISKS OF SMOKING MARIJUANA

One of my patients, Beth, sixteen, smoked pot several times a week. Her mom knew about it but was afraid if she told Beth to stop, it would make things worse. "Then she'd just do it behind my back," her mother told me.

I told Beth the facts about marijuana and encouraged her to quit.

"The health risks of smoking pot are the same as, maybe even greater than, those for smoking cigarettes. Smoking a joint can cause lung cancer, too," I told her.

I also talked to her about how marijuana works. I explained that marijuana, which comes from the cannabis plant, contains more than four hundred chemicals. Even though it's the most commonly used illegal substance in the United States—about 34 percent of high school girls have tried pot at least once[53]—it has all kinds of risks. In addition to the cancer risks that come from any kind of smoking, pot has a powerful effect on the brain. In the short term it might make you mellow or giddy. If you've ever known anyone who smokes a lot of marijuana, you've probably already noticed the long-term effects, which can include the loss of mental sharpness and focus.

Pot also poses another danger that cigarette smoking doesn't. Because it's an illegal substance, there are no rules and regulations making sure marijuana is pure and hasn't been tampered with. Sometimes marijuana is laced with other dangerous substances, such as PCP (angel dust), a dangerous hallucinogenic. There's absolutely no way to know what you're actually smoking. The one thing you do know for sure is that the pot was made and distributed by people breaking the law. Are those the folks you want deciding what you put in your body?

I don't know if my advice sank in with Beth. But at least she heard the facts from a doctor and had the chance to make her own choice.

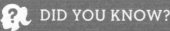

DID YOU KNOW?
Fewer Teens Are Smoking Pot

The number of high school students smoking marijuana is dropping. In 1999 nearly half of high school students had tried pot. Today that's dropped to 38 percent of all high schoolers, and just 34 percent of girls.[54] That's great news.

ASK YOURSELF: PEER PRESSURE

I'm the first to admit I don't have all the answers. But you might. Ask yourself these questions—about yourself and about peer pressure in general. Your answers might help you feel stronger and more powerful the next time you're feeling pressured.

1. If I give in to the pressure to [smoke pot, smoke cigarettes, drink, have sex], what positive result would I be looking for? Acceptance, approval, more friends? Happiness?
2. Would this behavior actually get me the results I really want?
3. What other results—positive or negative—might it get me?

DR. ASHTON'S MAD SCIENTIST PLAYLIST

If you're curious about smoking, drinking, drugs, sex, or other risky behavior, you're not alone. In some ways experimenting is exactly what you're *supposed* to be doing as a teenager. This is the time when, psychologically, you're programmed to push the boundaries. But I tell my patients to choose their experiments wisely. As any scientist knows, some test tubes blow up in your face. Here's some other advice I share:

1. Experimentation is part of growing up—but you can skip certain experiments. You don't have to experiment with drinking, drugs, smoking, or other high-risk behaviors to have a healthy, normal teen experience.
2. If you feel the need to experiment, try a new haircut or fashion trend. They can't kill you—alcohol, drugs, and cigarettes can.

THINK, DON'T DRINK

Early one morning I got an emergency call from a mom, referred by a longtime patient of mine. The mom wanted me to examine her daughter, Stephanie, right away: Something terrible had happened the night before.

Stephanie's dad had dropped her off at a friend's Sweet Sixteen party. Stephanie said people at the party were drinking, but she wasn't. She stuck to the punch instead. She left the party around 11 p.m., when a friend's mother picked them up and brought them back to the friend's house for a sleepover. That's the last thing Stephanie remembers.

At 2:15 a.m. Stephanie's mom got a call from the doorman in their apartment building: Stephanie was passed out in the mailroom, in a pool of vomit, with her skirt up around her waist. They brought her to me to find out if Stephanie had been sexually attacked and to test her for sexually transmitted infections. I wasn't able to find any evidence of attack (this isn't always as easy and clear as you'd think), but at least her STI tests came back clean.

To this day we still don't know for sure what happened to Stephanie while she was unconscious. Our best guess is that the punch was spiked with alcohol or a date-rape drug and she blacked out. We'll never know exactly what took place, but we're all grateful that Stephanie made it home in one piece and didn't become a tragic statistic while she was blacked out.

To me Stephanie's story shows the huge dangers of teen drinking. Even though she wasn't drinking herself, simply being in an environment where teens were consuming alcohol placed her in an incredibly risky situation. Somebody wasn't using their best judgment or their conscience when they spiked her drink. Even if you're not a drinker, hanging out in high-risk environments, with people who are taking risks, means you're putting yourself in the way of other people's worst impulses.

MIXED MESSAGES

Alcohol is a funny substance, surrounded by double standards. It's socially and legally acceptable at some times in your life but not others. It's against the law until age twenty-one but legal for adults. In small amounts it's not harmful to your health, but in excess it can kill you. Your parents tell you never, ever to drink as a teen—but if you do, call them for a ride home. Talk about mixed messages. As with everything else, I believe knowledge is power. You're less likely to abuse alcohol if you understand how it works.

YOUR BRAIN ON ALCOHOL

When you drink an alcoholic beverage, your body starts to absorb the alcohol from your stomach into your bloodstream in as little as five to ten minutes. As soon as alcohol hits your brain, your body's central nervous system (the machinery that runs your body) starts to slow down. Your physical actions happen more slowly and your movements become a little sloppy. Your brain's circuitry doesn't fire as effectively, so thoughts and speech become impaired. Your judgment gets skewed, so you might say things that you wouldn't normally say or do things that you wouldn't normally do.

Your body can only metabolize a certain amount of alcohol in a certain amount of time. If you exceed that limit, your body shuts down important functions—like, say, breathing. Your respiratory rate slows down, and your blood gets less oxygen. Your stomach (wisely) wants to get rid of the toxins, so you may vomit. Unfortunately, if you're passed out at the time, you could easily choke on the vomit. If this happens, it's very likely you'll die.

Every single year teens and college students across the country die of alcohol poisoning. That's why you need to avoid drinking until you're twenty-one, and then drink only in moderation—never more than two drinks a night. You also need to be able to recognize signs of alcohol poisoning if you see it. (Read the box on page 256.) Watch out for your friends: Don't risk their lives.

If you do realize that someone you know is suffering from alcohol poisoning, forget what you've heard about black coffee and cold showers. They don't work.

Alcohol poisoning requires medical treatment. If a friend has signs of alcohol poisoning, alert an adult or call 911. Do not leave that person alone. Do not try to spare them embarrassment or keep them out of trouble: Save their life instead.

SIGNS OF ALCOHOL POISONING

Mental confusion

Slow or shallow breathing

Irregular breathing

Pale or blue-colored skin

Vomiting

Seizures

Inability to respond to shaking or commands

BRAIN POISON FOR TEENS

Medically speaking, even small amounts of alcohol are *not* OK for teens. Because teen brains are still developing, they're much more susceptible to potentially addictive substances and behaviors than adult brains. Drinking as a teen does far more damage to your brain than drinking in your twenties or later. Recent studies have shown that people who use drugs or alcohol before age fifteen were two to three times more likely to have addiction or dependence problems later in life. These same studies showed this group had higher rates of STIs, of dropping out of school, of criminal records, and of teen pregnancies. Overall this means that drinking as a teen isn't bad just for your health but for your future.

 DR. ASHTON'S ALCOHOL PLAYLIST

- You'll have your whole life to enjoy alcohol responsibly. You don't need to drink as a teen. Wait until your brain has developed enough to handle moderate drinking without damage.

READY, SET, NO

My friend Maggie always calls herself the "milk and cookies" type. In high school she was always ready for adventure—whether that was trying out for a school musical, checking out a new dance club, or learning to snowboard. But one thing she never felt adventurous about was drinking.

"It actually scared me," she said. "I always ended up feeling like some kind of wimp. But I didn't want to drink and I didn't like seeing my friends drunk. I'd rather go home and bake cookies. For a while I felt like a total loser, since I wasn't hanging out with my friends. But I came up with some good excuses so I could go out with them, have fun, and leave when they started drinking."

She ended up telling her friends that she couldn't drink because she was lacking an enzyme that digests alcohol. "I said even one drink could kill me," she recalls. And she'd volunteer to drive her friends home if they drank too much.

I think it's a very smart strategy to know exactly how you'll say no in any given situation. Armed with a ready-made excuse that you've practiced in the mirror a few times, you'll sound cool, confident, and totally in control. See my list of suggestions.

KNOW HOW TO SAY NO

With a little creativity, you can make most of these excuses fit any situation where you want to say no—drinking, drugs, sex, you name it.

1. "I don't believe in polluting my body."
2. "I just don't feel the need to experience altered consciousness. My own consciousness is just fine, thanks."
3. "I'd rather spend my calories on cookies."
4. "Didn't you hear about the teen who died from drinking during rush at his fraternity?"
5. "I'm missing the enzyme that digests alcohol. Even one drink could kill me."
6. "I have asthma and can't smoke."
7. "My parents do random drug testing at home."
8. "I'm afraid. If you tease me for that, I won't be your friend anymore."
9. "I'm driving tonight."

BAD THINGS HAPPEN WHEN YOU'RE DRUNK

Ever said anything you really regretted later? Done anything that made you feel like an idiot? Remember that miserable mortified feeling that made you wish you'd never been born?

Getting drunk is like volunteering to feel that way all over again. It's hard enough to say and do the right thing when you're sober. When you drink you're much, much more likely to use poor judgment. And I'm not talking about spilling the beans about your best friend's secret crush. (Though slips like that can happen all too easily, too, after even one drink.) I'm talking about putting yourself in risky situations—getting in a car with someone who's been drinking, making out with someone you don't know, trying drugs, or other risky behaviors. When you're drunk, some things can seem like good ideas—even when they're really, really bad ideas. Like one guy I went to school with. He got drunk at a party one night, went wandering around with friends, and ended up climbing on top of a train at the campus train station. He grabbed a wire overhead to steady himself. The electric shock didn't kill him, but he lost both of his legs. Stories like this happen every year. And not just to dumb people. To smart, fun, together people who happened to drink too much one night and will regret it the rest of their lives.

Something else to consider: Alcohol is associated with higher levels of violence. When you're around people who are drinking, their judgment is impaired, too, and they may be more likely to act violently or hurt you. If you're also drinking, you may be less able to defend yourself and more vulnerable. If you're sober, it's easier to extract yourself from risky situations.

The best way to avoid becoming a tragic statistic is to skip alcohol in your teens—and to avoid becoming drunk at any age.

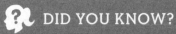

DID YOU KNOW?
Drinking and Driving Is a Major Cause of Teen Deaths

Motor vehicle accidents—many of which involve alcohol—are the single leading cause of death in people ages fifteen to twenty. In 2007 more than 1,800 people under twenty died in alcohol related motor vehicle accidents.[55]

DATE-RAPE DRUGS: IT HAPPENED TO ME

Here's another bad thing that can happen when you consume alcohol: You're more vulnerable to predators who spike drinks with so-called date-rape drugs. Sedatives and mind-altering drugs like GHB have no color, no odor, and no flavor. They render you unable to speak, walk, defend yourself, or remember what happened. This isn't an urban myth. It really happens. I know because it happened to me.

I was a senior in college at Columbia University in New York City, working as a bartender in a very hot bar. I wasn't much of a drinker in high school or college, but I liked bartending. I got to enjoy the party atmosphere without drinking—and while earning good money.

One night a bunch of local college students came in celebrating a big football win. A very cute guy offered to buy me a beer (we bartenders were all over twenty-one, so the boss let us drink a little—only a little—while working). I rarely drank, but it was a really fun night and I got caught up in the moment. I poured myself a draft beer and took a few sips as I continued to tend the bar.

I never even finished half the beer. Before I knew it, I was in the basement stockroom, unable to stand and barely able to talk. I called my ex-boyfriend and couldn't say anything except his name. Knowing something was terribly wrong, he came over to find me passed out with absolutely no recollection of anything after the phone call. Someone had slipped me a "date-rape" drug. Fortunately, no one had gotten me alone. I consider myself incredibly lucky.

So-called date-rape drugs like GHB, Ketamine, and Rohypnol cause blackouts and amnesia. They take effect very rapidly and have a strong potential for overdose, which can lead to death. If you think you might have been drugged, seek medical attention immediately. (Tip: These drugs can be detected in urine samples, so don't pee before going to the hospital.)

The moral of my story is: Be street smart. These drugs can be slipped into any beverage (although they're much more common in settings where people are drinking alcohol). If you drink in moderation, be aware that you're more vulnerable. And don't let anything you're drinking out of your sight.

DID YOU KNOW?
Most Rapes and Sexual Assaults
Aren't Committed by Strangers

Drinking and drugs impair your judgment—and the judgment of the guys you're hanging out with. Protect yourself by knowing the facts.

- 73 percent of sexual assaults are perpetrated by a friend, family member, or acquaintance.[56]
- One in eight high school girls reports being raped.[57]
- More than 50 percent of all date rapes take place at a house or apartment.
- 15 percent of date rapes occur in dorm rooms or parked cars.
- One of three women who have been raped were raped between the ages of twelve and seventeen.

ESCAPE DATE RAPE[58]

Keep yourself safe from date rape with these tips:

- Avoid alcohol.
- Don't drink anything that hasn't been poured in front of you.
- Avoid uncomfortable or isolated situations.
- Don't hesitate to verbalize your feelings: If you don't like or want something, say so.
- Take a self-defense class, such as karate or mixed martial arts.
- NEVER leave a bar or party with someone you don't know—no matter how nice he seems.

> ## OTHER GOOD REASONS NOT TO DRINK
>
> - It's illegal if you're under twenty-one.
> - One beer typically has 150 to 200 calories, the equivalent of two small chocolate chip cookies. These are empty calories that do nothing good for your body.
> - It's bad for your liver and your brain.
> - You've got a much higher chance of using poor judgment, getting injured, or putting yourself in danger.

ALCOHOLISM IN THE FAMILY

More than 9 million children[59] in this country have a parent with a drinking or drug problem. If alcoholism affects your family, I want to tell you a few things.

First, you did not cause your parent's drinking problem. It's not your fault and it's not something you can fix. But you can ask for help. Don't feel embarrassed to talk to your doctor or a close adult friend or relative. Asking for help is a sign of maturity. National groups, including Al-Anon and Alateen, exist specifically to help support the families of alcoholics and enable you to better understand this disease and its effects on you. Look up www.al-anon.org.

You also need to know that having an alcoholic parent puts you at greater risk for alcohol problems yourself. There's a genetic component to substance abuse. Scientists are trying to isolate addiction genes so new medications can be developed to treat these problems. But until hereditary causes are better understood, children of alcoholics need to realize they're at higher risk for the same problem and should be more aggressive about prevention.

DO YOU (OR SOMEONE YOU KNOW) DRINK TOO MUCH?

Alcoholism is a negative pattern of alcohol use that leads to other problems, including medical issues such as increased tolerance or withdrawal symptoms and social problems. The actual amount that you drink is irrelevant. If drinking any amount at all is causing problems, that's alcoholism.

Usually the process of developing a problem with alcohol goes through five steps:

1. Having access to alcohol.
2. Experimenting with alcohol, leading to regular use.
3. Drinking more and more often.
4. Becoming preoccupied with drinking and with getting drunk.
5. Only feeling normal when using alcohol. At this last step, risk-taking behavior usually starts and problems increase.

TRAPPED IN A CAGE?[60]
IDENTIFYING PROBLEMS WITH ALCOHOL

These four questions—called the CAGE questions—can help you identify if you have a drinking problem.

C—Have you felt you should **cut down** on the amount or frequency that you drink?

A—Have friends or relatives **annoyed** you with their comments about your drinking habit?

G—Have you felt **guilty** about your habit?

E—Have you ever felt like you needed a drink as an **eye-opener,** to steady your nerves, or get rid of a hangover?

If you answered yes to even one of these questions, please talk to an adult you trust about your drinking.

 QUIZ

Which Has the Most Alcohol?

A. Beer
B. Wine
C. Hard liquor

ANSWER: C. Hard liquor may be up to 50 percent alcohol. Beer is 3 to 5 percent, and wine is 9 to 16 percent.

 DID YOU KNOW?
Two Drinks Might Be Too Many[61]

In every state it's illegal to drink if you're under twenty-one.[62] It's also illegal to drive in every state if your blood alcohol content is more than .08 percent.[63] If you're a 120-pound woman and have two drinks, you'll be at the limit. If you're 100 pounds, you can't have more than one drink and still be safe to drive.

If you feel a friend or someone you know has a problem with alcohol, immediately talk to another adult you trust—a friend, relative, or doctor. And if you suspect that you have a problem with alcohol, tell your parents right away. They need to know what's going on. If you absolutely can't do that, tell another adult you trust.

Next, get professional help from a psychologist, psychiatrist, or substance-abuse physician. Some teens need to be hospitalized or admitted to rehab to treat the disease. Some prescription medications might help: These work by producing a very unpleasant physical reaction when combined with alcohol. It's not easy to stop drinking when you're addicted. But the sooner you realize you have a problem, the better.

BE STREET SMART ABOUT STREET DRUGS

If you think all drug users are gang members, rock stars, pro athletes, or homeless people, guess again. Hard-drug users are also suburban housewives, doctors, movie stars, and even high school students, like my patient Leslie. Smart and pretty, Leslie tried cocaine at age sixteen when her friends talked her into it. She soon found she couldn't get enough. She became obsessed with her next hit, with getting more drugs, and hiding them from her parents.

Fortunately, Leslie got into rehab and has been clean and sober for two years. She told me she feels incredibly lucky that she never got arrested, assaulted, or raped. In fact, she feels lucky just to be alive.

As Leslie found out, street drugs are pervasive. You can find them in small towns, big cities, and everywhere in between.

Here's what they do to your body and mind.

Cocaine. Also known as "coke," "blow," "snow," or "C." Made from the coca bush, cocaine can be very addictive (natural isn't always safe!). It works rapidly on the heart and the brain.

In the brain cocaine alters the perception of feelings of pleasure, reality, and mood. Over the long term people who use cocaine often suffer from depression and display generally self-destructive tendencies. Cocaine also causes a very rapid heart rate, elevates blood pressure, and increases body temperature. At times these abnormal heart rates are fatal. With cocaine your first time could easily be your last.

Ecstasy. Also known as X. This is an amphetamine or "upper" that causes psychedelic changes in your emotional and sensory perception.

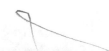

About 5.8 percent of high school students[64] have tried ecstasy. The technical term for this drug is MDMA, but I just call it really bad news. Despite its cheerful name, ecstasy has potentially devastating neurotoxic effects. In the long run, it can permanently damage your brain and central nervous system. In the short term, ecstasy can cause dehydration and can cross-react with other drugs, leading to death.

Heroin. Made from morphine, which comes from opium derived from the poppy plant. (Remember in the *Wizard of Oz* when Dorothy falls asleep in the poppy field?) When heroin hits your bloodstream, it goes directly to the brain, where it has a sedative effect. It can also impair important bodily functions like breathing. In terms of feelings and sensations, heroin acts like a powerful narcotic (painkiller) and slows down your thoughts and reactions. Heroin is highly addictive and associated with several other very serious health risks, such as hepatitis C and HIV/AIDS. The overall use and abuse of heroin is on the rise in the United States.

Crystal Meth. Another form of stimulant or amphetamine. Often called ice, it's clear, odorless, and tasteless. Crystal meth works a lot like cocaine, but the effects last longer and are much more extreme. In the short term, it can cause suicidal, homicidal or violent thoughts, and paranoia and anxiety. Physically, crystal meth increases heart rate and blood pressure, which can lead to seizures and death. Continued use can cause serious effects in the brain, resulting in symptoms similar to those of Parkinson's disease, Alzheimer's disease, and general brain damage.

PRESCRIPTION DRUGS

Over the past few years we've heard more and more about prescription drug use as a source of serious problems for teens. At one end of the spectrum is sneaking prescription medications from your parents' medicine cabinet. At the other end there's "pharming." Possibly an urban legend, but one that clearly illustrates the dangers of prescription drugs, the story goes like this: You show up at a party and find a giant bowl filled with random pills. People pass it around like a big bowl of popcorn, dig their hands in, and swallow fistfuls of unknown prescription drugs. Where did they come from? Parents' medicine cabinets—their antidepressants or anxiety medicines, sleeping pills, painkillers, high blood pressure medications, even hormones.

At both ends of the spectrum, abusing prescription drugs is every bit as dangerous and potentially deadly as buying cocaine off the street. Anytime you're taking unknown pills—whether from your own bathroom or the party punch bowl—you're taking a huge risk. You have no idea what you're taking. Even if you do know, you probably don't have a clue how one drug might interact with another, or how strong they are. You don't know the possible side effects, dangers, or other risks involved.

Never, never risk your life by popping a handful of prescription medications or raiding your parents' medicine chest. Even one pill might be enough to put you into a coma. And repeatedly taking prescription medications can lead to physical dependence or addiction.

"DRUG ABUSE, AISLE TWO"

Just because something's for sale at the drugstore doesn't mean it's safe. In fact, anything sold on the drug aisle is potentially deadly in excessive amounts. That goes for aspirin, Tylenol, Motrin, Bengay muscle rub, Pepto-Bismol, Midol, Benadryl, you name it. Those instructions on the package are there for a reason. Never take more than the directed amount or take it more often than recommended on the package, unless a doctor tells you to. Otherwise you could harm your liver, your kidneys, or your brain.

If you're feeling bad enough to cruise the aisles of your local drugstore looking for an over-the-counter remedy, you deserve to feel better. Tell your parents, talk to your doctor, or find other adults you can trust.

DID YOU KNOW?
Common Medicines Can Kill You

- Cough medicine/cold remedies: Contain a drug called DXM, which is very similar to morphine. Excess use can cause respiratory problems, coma, or death.
- Weight-loss aids: Many contain ephedrine or pseudoephedrine, a powerful stimulant. Excess use can cause dangerously rapid heart rate or fatal cardiac arrhythmia.
- Motion-sickness pills: Taken in excess amounts, these can cause drowsiness and hallucinations or even death.

KILLING THE BUZZ

OK, so this chapter was a total buzz-kill. That's the whole point: I want you to know the sobering truth about drinking, drugs, smoking, and other high-risk behaviors so you'll make better choices. I can't stop you from trying any of these. Neither can your parents. It's your life, it's your body, it's your decision.

But I *can* give you the facts to help you make informed choices—and I hope you'll base your decisions on facts, not peer pressure or insecurity. If I can help you do that, then I'm definitely willing to be a buzz-kill. Especially if it keeps you from getting killed.

CHAPTER 13

BLUE IS *NOT* YOUR COLOR

Managing Moods and Mood Disorders

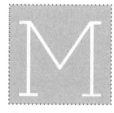y patient Theresa had warm, chocolate-brown eyes, loved music, and had a singing voice like Beyoncé. I started treating her when she was in tenth grade. She went off to college and came back to see me about halfway through her freshman year for a routine exam. I thought her energy seemed a little low, but her exam showed she was fine. Physically, anyway.

"So what else is going on with you? How's school?" I asked at the end of the visit. It's a routine question: I try to understand what's going on in my patients' lives—one, because it's really interesting, and two, because health issues aren't just about physical symptoms. All kinds of things in your life can influence your physical and mental health, so I need to know the big picture.

In Theresa's case, my ordinary question sparked a far-from-ordinary response. She suddenly started crying and told me she'd been sad, lonely, and struggling with her classes for months. When she said she'd even quit her singing lessons, I knew something was very wrong.

"That sounds really serious," I said.

"It's been bad. Actually . . ." she paused, then rushed on, "I was so miserable I was thinking about hurting myself."

Fortunately, Theresa's roommate insisted on taking her to the campus counseling center. Realizing that Theresa was suicidal, a psychiatrist had her admitted to a hospital near campus where she could be safely cared for. She started taking medication and her parents came to take her home. Now she'd been home for about a week.

"OK, so what's the plan? What happens next?" I asked.

Theresa shrugged. It turned out there *was* no plan. No one had made her any follow-up appointments with therapists or psychiatrists. I was alarmed, and I called a friend of mine who's a terrific psychiatrist. We got Theresa an appointment a few days later.

It turned out Theresa was suffering from clinical depression. It wasn't simply that she was sad about something in particular. She just couldn't cheer herself up no matter how hard she tried.

The good news is, depression is one of the most common and most treatable of mental disorders. Theresa eventually found a good mix of "talk therapy" and antidepressant medication that helped her feel like her normal self. Now she's singing again and applying to graduate school to be a music teacher. Along the way, she's learned a lot about managing the physical disease of depression.

THE MIND-BODY CONNECTION

So what's a nice gynecologist like me doing in a mood chapter like this? I'm definitely *not* a psychiatrist or psychologist. But anyone who works closely with teen girls knows that emotional health is critical to physical health. How your mind and heart feel affects how your body feels—and vice versa.

Your mental state can also affect the choices you make and how you take care of yourself. Small example: When you're in a blue mood, you might not feel like exercising—and not exercising can make you even *more* depressed. Big example: Some girls with mood problems try to self-medicate and experiment with drinking and other risky behavior. To take the best possible care of yourself, you need to understand the role that moods play in your health. And you need to understand when you can help yourself feel better—and when you need professional help to start feeling as good as you deserve.

JUST A BAD DAY? OR A MOOD DISORDER?

We all get in a bad mood sometimes (I sure do—just ask my family!). But most of the time we get over it. The good news is, as you become more mature, you also get smarter about what helps you get *out* of a bad mood. One patient of mine realized that she got bitchy whenever she stopped exercising—now she makes a point to get to the gym five days a week. Another patient discovered that when she's doing yoga regularly she's more patient with herself and her family. Some of my patients go to a movie, escape into a book, or listen to their iPods. Even if none of our usual tricks work, most of us know that sooner or later something will snap us back into our normal happy selves.

But people with mood disorders *can't* help themselves feel normal. Their blues aren't something the Jonas Brothers or a few old episodes of *Gilmore Girls* can cure. Instead people with mood disorders have a biological condition that they truly can't treat themselves. Two of the most common mood disorders are depression and bipolar disorder (where depression alternates with out-of-control elation).

Mood disorders are one kind of mental disorder—a category that also includes eating disorders (see chapter 10), social phobias, anxiety disorder, and obsessive-compulsive disorder. So, technically, if you have depression, you have a mental disorder. But that does *not* mean you're crazy. It means your body's not working right. Specifically researchers think mental illnesses, including mood disorders, result from chemical imbalances in the brain. It's not your fault if you have one. And it's great if you realize that you have symptoms, because fortunately mood disorders (and most mental illnesses in general) are treatable. And the sooner you start treating them, the better.

Whether you have a mental disorder or just a case of the normal blues, it's important to understand what's normal and what isn't, and how to find help.

 DID YOU KNOW?
More Than One in Ten Teens Get Major Depression

Major depressive episodes—times of severe, persistent depression, sometimes with loss of appetite, exhaustion, lethargy, sleep problems, or thoughts of self-harm—are surprisingly common in teens.[65]

- In 2005, 3-4 million youths ages twelve to seventeen had at least one major depressive episode. That's 13.7 percent of the youth population.
- Girls are more likely to have major depressive episodes than boys. About 13.3 percent of girls ages twelve to seventeen have had one, compared with 4.5 percent of boys.
- Having a major depressive episode is associated with higher rates of drug or alcohol problems—19.8 percent of youths who had major depressive episodes have had a problem with illegal substances, including alcohol.

DR. ASHTON'S MOODY BLUES PLAYLIST

- Depression is a disease, like high blood pressure. Don't be embarrassed to have it, and please don't think it's a personal shortcoming.
- You're not alone. One in ten American teens and children suffer from a mental illness significant enough to affect their day-to-day life.
- Mood disorders are not all in your head. You can't think your way out with a positive mental attitude. You need help. Seeking out help shows how mature you are.

WHAT'S NORMAL, WHAT'S NOT

Everyday "blues" are like the common cold—everybody gets them, and you'll shake them sooner or later, especially if your sadness comes from something specific, like breaking up with your boyfriend or fighting with your BFF.

Clinical depression, on the other hand, is a major disease and often won't just go away on its own.

So how do you know the difference? One way is to look at your life. Major stress events often lead to some degree of sadness, anger, or unhappiness. It's perfectly normal to feel a little off if you've had a big fight with your best friend or if your parents are getting divorced.

That's why doctors want to know what's going on in your life, especially if you're showing signs of depression. If you were an adult and told a doctor you were feeling down, the first thing he or she would do is look at the list of major life stress events.

ADULT STRESS EVENTS

Getting married

Starting a job

Moving

Having a baby

Death of a spouse, child, or parent

Getting divorced

Notice that not all these things are bad! Getting married, starting a new job, having a baby—these are all pretty exciting in a good way. But *any* big life change can throw you off. When adults experience one of these events, their doctors wouldn't be surprised or alarmed to hear that they're feeling stressed, overwhelmed, sad, or anxious.

But guess what? There's no official list for teens! If I had to write my own list, here's what I'd include. I bet you can think of more.

MAJOR STRESS EVENTS FOR TEENS

Changing schools

Breaking up with a girlfriend or boyfriend

Going to college

Death of a parent, sibling, or friend

Experiencing a major illness or accident

Divorce of parents

Major rejection by a best friend or peer group

You get the point: Adolescence can be seriously stressful.

Everybody deals with stress like this in different ways. Some teens slam doors or scream at their parents or cry for days. Others shut themselves up in their rooms. Any of this can potentially be normal, but occasionally reactions veer off track into extreme behaviors that aren't considered normal—like smashing a vase or breaking a window with a baseball bat. Extreme reactions hint that something's not quite right.

LEARNING TO COPE

As a young girl you're evolving rapidly into an adult—which means experiencing a new range of emotions. Learning to deal with these emotions is a vital skill that you'll use for the rest of your life. You learn coping strategies from family and friends and also by trial and error. Here are some strategies that my patients use to cope with stress—they might help you, too.

- **Writing in a journal:** Studies show that people who write about their deep emotions and about stressful events have better health than those who don't.[66]
- **Exercising:** One study at Duke University found that walking or jogging for thirty minutes three times a week helped reduce depression as much as taking medication.[67]
- **Listening to music:** Studies show listening to relaxing music can reduce stress for surgery patients, pregnant moms, and other groups. It may help you, too.
- **Talking with friends or family:** Don't bottle up your feelings. Talking about your problems may make you feel much better. But if it *doesn't* make you feel better, don't push it or dwell on things at length. One study found that girls who spent an excessive amount of time talking about their problems with friends actually felt worse.[68]
- **Healthy eating:** Some foods, vitamins, and good eating habits may boost your mood. (See page 281-83 for details.)

If you've tried all your usual tricks and you're still not feeling better, you may have a mood disorder.

NO SHAME, NO BLAME: THE 411 ON MENTAL DISORDERS

Scientists are only beginning to understand what causes mental illnesses in teens.

One thing we do know is that mental illness runs in families, so if you have a family member with a mental disorder, you're at risk, too.

Environment also plays a role in mental illness. If your family or social environments are unusually difficult or stressful or include drug or alcohol abuse or violence, you're more likely to experience mood disorders. Stressful events like the death of a loved one or parents getting divorced might cause short-term sorrow . . . but they can also lead to deep and prolonged depression that requires treatment.

Finally, medical conditions like thyroid problems and cancer can cause or worsen depression or mood disorders—and so can some medications (like heart medications, some hormones, or blood pressure medications). If you take any prescriptions or herbal therapies and notice a change in your mood, tell your doctor right away.

MENTAL ILLNESS FACTORS

- Family history/genetics
- Family or social environment
- Life events
- Medications or medical conditions

Here's a quick overview of the three most common mood disorders in teens. If you or someone you know has any of the signs, please talk to a doctor or another adult you trust right away.

DEPRESSION

True depression isn't just feeling sad—it's a partial or total transformation of your personality. Sadness, hopelessness, and despair flood your life and affect your every thought and action. If you're clinically depressed, you might cry all the time or constantly feel anxious. You might withdraw from your family and friends, stop enjoying your usual activities, have trouble sleeping or eating, or even think about suicide or hurting yourself. Most teens feel some of these things some of the time, but the feelings pass fairly soon. But true depression doesn't go away on its own.

SIGNS OF DEPRESSION

- Deep sadness, despair, guilt, or hopelessness
- Eating too much or too little
- Insomnia or excessive sleeping
- Trouble concentrating
- Withdrawing from friends and family
- Tearfulness and crying
- Irritability, anger, or anxiety
- Thoughts of death or suicide

Usually depression appears in teens around age fifteen. It's twice as likely to affect girls as boys, since girls are more likely to internalize depressive feelings. Internalizing feelings doesn't mean you never talk about your emotions. It means you take thoughts or feelings to a deeper level and harness them emotionally rather than physically. Boys who feel sad or depressed are more likely to act out—through fights, drug or alcohol use, or defiant behavior.

It's easy for adults to miss depression in teens. After all, many parents *expect* teens to be moody or behave erratically sometimes. Plus, a depressed teen might be so difficult to be around that adults closest to her might not see the signs. And teen depression symptoms aren't identical to adult depression signs. Some depressed adults simply curl up in bed and stop functioning; teens usually have to keep getting up and going to school, so they're forced to keep functioning, sort of. And depressed teens sometimes rally and go out with friends. This all makes it hard for parents to believe their daughter is depressed: "But she still goes out with her friends," parents tell me. In fact, it's so easy to miss depression in teens that some experts say less than half of adolescents with depression receive any treatment.

BIPOLAR DISORDER

As if being depressed weren't hard enough, people with bipolar disorder also experience manic periods—times of extreme energy, racing thoughts, and an irrationally elated mood. Depression doesn't always come with mania—but mania *always* comes with depression. It's impossible to have it alone: Sooner or later depression will set in.

Some specialists think bipolar disorder is overdiagnosed in teens and that their symptoms are actually a part of a borderline personality disorder (another type of mental condition). But there's no question that these extremes in mood do occur. This is a potentially very serious condition that often requires a lifetime of treatment to control.

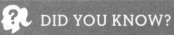

DID YOU KNOW?
ADD Can Masquerade as Bipolar Disorder

Some studies suggest that as many as 15 percent of children with bipolar disorder actually have attention deficit disorder (ADD) or attention deficit hyperactivity disorder (ADHD) and have been misdiagnosed.

Here's a disturbing trend thought to be on the rise among U.S. teens and preteens: self-inflicted cuts, burns, and scratches. Some experts think this is a way to cope with stress; others see it as a way to punish oneself; still others suggest it's a way to fit in with peers. Whatever the reason, sometimes girls repeatedly cut, burn, scratch, or even bite their arms or other body parts.

Studies have shown that girls who cut themselves are more likely to have difficulty expressing their emotions safely as adults. Sometimes people who injure themselves like this suffer from underlying depression or anxiety, obsessive-compulsive disorder, or post-traumatic stress disorder. If you or someone you know is cutting, please find help right away. Talk to an adult you trust about the problem. This behavior requires professional treatment.

HELP FOR MOOD DISORDERS

If you think you or a friend or family member might have depression or another mood disorder, tell someone—a parent, an adult friend, a teacher, or a doctor. If you don't tell someone, things probably will get worse, not better.

To diagnose a mood disorder, a doctor talks to you about your feelings and symptoms and does a physical exam to make sure it's not some other illness that's causing the problem. If your doctor thinks you're depressed or have another mood disorder, she or he may refer you for treatment to a counselor. Three kinds of professionals often work together to treat mental disorders:

Psychiatrists: Medical doctors (M.D.s) trained in psychiatric diseases who can prescribe medications and talk with their patients to explore their deep mental issues.

Psychologists: Ph.D.s (not medical doctors) who provide long-term "talk therapy," helping you explore your feelings and emotions. Psychologists can help you make a plan to change your behavior and reactions. Psychologists and psychiatrists often work together to provide long-term treatment for conditions like depression and bipolar disorder.

Social workers: These professionals usually have a master's degree and can help you deal with a wide variety of problems. A social worker can't prescribe medication or admit you to a hospital but can provide helpful advice and counseling for ongoing problems. Often social workers are good at hooking you up with helpful resources like support groups or programs dealing with specific issues (like dealing with divorce, coping with the death of a loved one, or other stressful events).

BACK TO YOUR OLD SELF: HELP FOR MOOD DISORDERS

If you gotta have a mood disorder, now is the time to do it. The world knows much more today about depression and other mood disorders than ever before and many treatments are available. Some are medications; others are therapies like those listed below. Often a combination of approaches works best. The important thing is to find a solution that works for you. Here are a few approaches that work for different situations.

Behavioral Therapy. This approach teaches you positive ways to change your behavior, react to events, and use better strategies to deal with your problems. It's a very practical approach: If one strategy doesn't help, the therapist should have lots of other tricks up her sleeve.

Expressive Therapy. This approach encourages you to express your emotions through art, music, dance, or writing. Drawing, painting, or other forms of creative expression can help you resolve inner conflicts and find new, safe ways to express your feelings. Research shows that sound or music therapy can increase blood flow and help release the body's own natural mood chemicals. And dance therapy in particular seems helpful for teens who've been physically or emotionally abused, because it gives them a sense of the power and strength of their bodies.

Guided Imagery/Visual Therapy. When I was studying to take my medical school entrance exams, I used mental imagery to boost my concentration when I studied and give me more confidence when I took the test. It was fun, easy, and very powerful. Basically, a therapist guides you in creating a mental image you associate with health, peace, and wellness. If you summon this image when you're feeling anxious, it can help calm you down. It worked for me—I got into med school! But it also works for more severe anxiety and phobias.

FEELING YOUR FOOD

Some scientists call your guts and intestines your "second brain." That's because there's a powerful connection between what you eat and how you feel and act. Just think of how awful you feel when you skip a meal. And how good it feels to reach for a pint of Ben and Jerry's (or your own personal comfort food) after a huge fight with your mom. There's actually some truth to the rumor that chocolate boosts your mood—and some other foods may help even more.

While no therapist will recommend reaching for junk food to soothe your mood—and neither do I (see chapter 11)—there are some *healthy* dietary changes your therapist might recommend if you're being treated for a mood disorder. Even if you don't have a mood disorder, you might find that boosting some of these foods helps you manage your normal bad moods a little bit better.

Vitamin D

Vitamin D, which you can get from salmon and fortified milk—and also sunlight—is related to the production of serotonin, a substance in the brain that helps regulate mood. Too little D equals too little serotonin equals depression. You can boost your vitamin D intake with supplements of up to 1000 units a day.

More could be dangerous, so check with your doctor before taking larger doses.

Omega-3 Fatty Acids

Like vitamin D, omega-3 fatty acids also are vital for the function of serotonin and other neurotransmitters. Natural sources of omega-3 fatty acids include nuts, fish, and omega-3–fortified eggs.

Soluble Fiber

You've probably heard that fiber's good for your digestive tract. But it's also great for stabilizing your blood sugar levels. If your blood glucose levels stay steady throughout the day, you'll feel better. Good sources of fiber include oatmeal, fruits and veggies, brown rice, and whole wheat pastas and breads. Whole bran is good, too—but skip the sweet, sticky bran muffins and choose something lower in sugar and fat instead.

Caffeine

Caffeine's merits seem to shift with the weather. One day it's great for you; the next everybody says you should quit completely. The truth is that medicine, like life, is rarely black or white. Too much caffeine is clearly bad for you and carries real health risks. But in moderation caffeine can be good for your body and your mood. Studies have shown that small amounts of caffeine can increase mental function and improve sharpness, focus, and mood. But skip the Red Bulls and other energy drinks, sodas, and sweetened teas. Instead go for healthier sources like black tea, coffee, or dark chocolate.

B Vitamins

The B complex vitamins, including folate, are also very important for good mental health. A recent Harvard study found that almost 40 percent of depressed women were deficient in folate! Natural sources include nuts, brown rice, avocados (bring on the guacamole!), fish, and veggies. If you're on birth control pills or—ironically—antidepressants, you may suffer from a B complex deficiency—which could be contributing to your depression. Taking a B complex supplement may help.

DON'T WORRY, BE HAPPY

I want you to feel great physically, mentally, and emotionally—and those three areas are all connected. If you feel you're overly sad, depressed, angry, panicked, or anxious about events or your life in general, or if you're just not feeling like yourself, *please* speak to someone about your concerns. Asking for help is not a sign of weakness. In fact, reaching out for help is a sign of courage, maturity, and strength. And it's the first step toward feeling great.

CONCLUSION: THE GREATEST JOB IN THE WORLD

I've told you throughout this book how much I love my job. Taking care of teens like you and helping you become a strong, healthy, powerful woman who knows how to take care of herself, for life, is the most rewarding job I can possibly imagine.

But there's only so far I can take it. My work is done here, and now it's your job to put all this information into action. You've read the book, you know the facts. Only you can make smart choices for your body. Sometimes it will be easy and feel great. Sometimes it might seem like a drag or a lot of work—finding the time to exercise in your already crazed schedule, summoning the strength to choose the apple over the candy bar, explaining to your boyfriend—yet again—that you're waiting until at least eighteen for sex.

But the payoff is huge. Make good choices now, and you won't just survive junior high and high school. You'll thrive. You'll feel and look your best. You'll stay healthy. And, most important, as you make smart choices and stick with tough decisions, you'll learn to respect and value yourself. Nobody can give you the key to happiness. But learn these lessons now—about taking care of yourself, making smart choices, and valuing your body and your mind—and I promise you, you'll be on the road to becoming the smart, beautiful, healthy, powerful woman you hope to be and deserve to be. Not just now, but for the rest of your life. And what job—even mine—could be better than that?

ACKNOWLEDGMENTS

This book was easy to write. It was easy because it represents what I do every day—talk to teenage girls and help them grow into the strong, healthy women of tomorrow. It was not easy, however, to get this book published, and for that there are many people without whom that accomplishment would not have been possible. These individuals shared my dream of creating a book that would serve as the definitive guide for teenage girls for years to come, and for that they have my deepest appreciation and gratitude.

To begin, my love of writing was fostered and formally molded at the Horace Mann School over three years in English class with the late Edward Simpson. My medical mentors, Dr. Lisa Anderson and Dr. Daniel Stein, were among the few physicians who encouraged me to pursue my interest in adolescent gynecology. This interest was further supported by joining the North American Society of Pediatric and Adolescent Gynecology and by attending terrific presentations by Dr. Dianne Merritt, Dr. Jonathan Trager, and many other adolescent gynecologists at the society's yearly clinical meetings. I am also grateful to psychiatrist Dr. Allegra Broft for her assistance with the chapter on eating disorders, and to psychologist Dr. Linda Centeno for reviewing the chapter on mood disorders.

Outside the medical world, Richard C. Auletta believed in me enough to introduce me to my literary agent, David Hale Smith, himself a father of two young girls. David "got it." He saw the need for this book, not just for his daughters, but for adolescent girls everywhere. Christine Larson, my collaborator, exemplified the term "professional writer" and made the transition of thought to word seem effortless. My literary attorney, Robert Stein, and my editor, Lucia Watson at Avery/Penguin, were invaluable in facilitating the process. My agent, Kenneth Slotnick, and his team at William Morris Endeavor Entertainment, has been exceptional in his insight and support. In making the cover expressive of the relatable nature of the book, and in helping me (as the messenger of a very important message) deliver this communication visually, I am extremely grateful to photographer Michael Benabib, makeup artist extraordinaire Mario Dedivanovic, and hair stylist Jeanna Mirante. The clothing for the cover was supplied by Hamrah's of NJ.

Inside *my* world, my friends and family provided indefatigable support and encouragement for this project. My dear friend Dr. Mehmet Oz has served as unofficial book adviser and role model. Kathy Leventhal (former publisher of *Allure* magazine) gave this project a publisher's eye and a mother's heart. Gerette Allegra understood the importance of *The Body Scoop* from the moment I described it to her. My "teen consultants" Hannah Sutker and my goddaughter Zoë Oz read rough drafts and gave me their fresh teen perspectives. The team at my private medical practice, Hygeia Gynecology, Ana Olivera and Carole Gittleman, share my dedication to the care of teen patients. And for encouraging me during the early days of my writing the book, I thank the labor and delivery nurses at Englewood Hospital and Medical Center.

Without the love and support of my parents, Dorothy Garfein and Dr. Oscar Garfein, my aunt and fellow ob-gyn, Dr. Barbara McCormack, and my family, this book would not have had the attention it required. My husband, Dr. Robert Ashton, never doubted the importance of *The Body Scoop* or the ability to make this book a reality, not only for our daughter, but for daughters everywhere. My children, Alex and Chloë, who participated in the writing and editing of the book, share my excitement regarding its completion.

Finally, I dedicate this book to my teenage patients and thank them from the bottom of my heart for the privilege of being their doctor. I admire their strength, adore their personalities, and appreciate the intelligence with which they approach their bodies and their health. Taking care of them provides me with endless inspiration and gratification. This special doctor-patient relationship is truly a two-way street: They give me the "scoop" on teenage life, and I give them the "scoop" on their bodies, their health, and their wellness. Now *that's* a partnership!

NOTES

1. Like all the girls I mention in this book, Casey is based on several of my real patients. However, all details have been modified and new composite characters have been created to protect my patients' confidentiality.
2. Steingraber, Sandra, "The Falling Age of Puberty in U.S. Girls." The Breast Cancer Fund, August 2007.
3. Klein, Jerry, and Iris Litt, "Epidemiology of Adolescent Dysmenorrhea." *Pediatrics*, November 1981.
4. Schroeder, B., and J. Sanfilippo, "Dysmenorrhea and Pelvic Pain in Adolescents." *Pediatric Clinics of North America*, June 1999.
5. Ibid.
6. Klein and Litt, "Epidemiology of Adolescent Dysmenorrhea."
7. Ibid.
8. Rapkin, Andrea, and Judith Mikacich, "Premenstrual Syndrome and Premenstrual Dysphoric Disorder in Adolescents." *Current Opinion in Obstetrics and Gynecology*, November 2008.
9. Ibid.
10. Braverman, Paula, M.D., Cincinnati Children's Hospital Medical Center lecture: Tattoos, Piercing and Body Modification in Teens, April 2008.
11. Unless otherwise noted, statistics in this chapter are from *Taking Care of Your "Girls": A Breast Health Guide for Girls, Teens, and In-Betweens* by Marisa Weiss, M.D., and Isabel Friedman (Three Rivers Press, 2008).
12. Sprague, et al., "Exercise and Breast Cancer." *British Medical Journal*, February 16, 2007.
13. Freidenreich, Christine, et al. Alberta Health Services—Alberta Cancer Board, 2009.
14. Ibid.
15. National Osteoporosis Foundation.
16. Institute of Medicine Daily Recommended Intake Elements Table: www.iom.edu.

17. Dietary Guidelines for Americans, 2005: www.health.gov.
18. Physical Activity and Health: A Report of the Surgeon General, 1996. Centers for Disease Control, National Center for Chronic Disease Prevention and Health Promotion.
19. Driscoll, D.A., "Polycystic Ovarian Syndrome in Adolescence." *Annals of the New York Academy of Science*, 2003.
20. Most of the statistics in this chapter, unless otherwise noted, come from the Guttmacher Institute: www.guttmacher.org.
21. U.S. Teen Sexual Activity. Kaiser Family Foundation, 2005.
22. "Virginity and the First Time." Kaiser Family Foundation, 2003.
23. "Reaching the MTV Generation." Kaiser Family Foundation, 2003.
24. "Virginity and the First Time." Kaiser Family Foundation, 2003.
25. "Sex Education in America: A Series of National Surveys of Students, Parents, Teachers and Principals." Kaiser Family Foundation, 2000.
26. Lindau, Stacy Tessler, et al., "What Schools Teach Our Patients About Sex." *Obstetrics and Gynecology*, February 2008.
27. Guttmacher Institute.
28. Statistics from the Wisconsin Coalition Against Sexual Assault: www.wicip.org.
29. Massey, J., "Domestic Violence in Neurological Practice." *Archives in Neurology*, 1999.
30. Effectiveness statistics from www.plannedparenthood.org.
31. "U.S. Teenage Pregnancy Statistics, National and State Trends and Trends by Race and Ethnicity." The Guttmacher Institute, 2006.
32. Jones, Rachel, et al., "Patterns in the Socioeconomic Characteristics of Women Obtaining Abortions in 2000-2001." *Perspectives on Sexual and Reproductive Health*, September/October 2002.
33. Most of the statistics on birth control methods come from Planned Parenthood: www.plannedparenthood.org.
34. "Trends in Reportable Sexually Transmitted Diseases in the United States." Centers for Disease Control, 2007.
35. Dunne, Eileen, et al., "Prevalence of HPV Infection Among Females in the United States." *Journal of the American Medical Association*, February 28, 2007.
36. Centers for Disease Control, 2007.
37. Ibid.
38. Menon, Seema, "Teens Lack Knowledge of STIs." Presented at the Annual Clinical Meeting, North American Society for Pediatrics and Adolescent Gynecology, July 2008.
39. Joint United Nations Programme on HIV/AIDS. 2008 Report on the Global AIDS Epidemic.

40. Herzog D.B., et al., "Mortality in Eating Disorders: A Descriptive Study." *International Journal of Eating Disorders*, 2000.

41. Ratey, John, *Spark: The Revolutionary New Science of Exercise and the Brain* (Little, Brown & Co., 2008).

42. Young, Lisa R., *The Portion Teller* (Broadway Books, 2005).

43. Zernike, Kate, "Sizing Up America: Signs of Expansion." *The New York Times*, March 1, 2004.

44. Substance Abuse and Mental Health Services Administration (2007). Results from the 2006 National Survey on Drug Use and Health. Office of Applied Studies.

45. National Institute on Drug Abuse.

46. "Second Hand Smoke Fact Sheet." American Lung Association.

47. "The Health Consequences of Smoking: A Report of the Surgeon General." Department of Health and Human Services, Centers for Disease Control and Prevention, National Center for Chronic Disease Prevention and Health Promotion, Office on Smoking and Health, 2004.

48. *Morbidity and Mortality Weekly Update*, June 26, 2008. Centers for Disease Control and Prevention. National Center for Chronic Disease Prevention and Health Promotion, Office on Smoking and Health.

49. "Preventing Tobacco Use Among Young People: A Report of the Surgeon General, 1994." Department of Health and Human Services, Centers for Disease Control and Prevention, National Center for Chronic Disease Prevention and Health Promotion, Office on Smoking and Health.

50. Saarni, Suoma, "Association of Smoking in Adolescence with Abdominal Obesity in Adulthood: A Follow-Up Study of Five Birth Cohorts of Finnish Twins." *American Journal of Public Health*, February 2009.

51. "The Health Consequences of Smoking."

52. Youth Risk Behavior Survey 2007. Centers for Disease Control.

53. Ibid.

54. "Trends in the Prevalence of Marijuana, Cocaine, and Other Illegal Drug Use National YRBS: 1991–2007." Youth Risk Behavior Survey 2007. Centers for Disease Control.

55. 2007 Traffic Safety Annual Assessment. Alcohol-Impaired Driving Fatalities. National Highway Traffic Safety Authority.

56. Rape, Abuse and Incest National Network.

57. Tool Kit for Teen Care, 2003. American College of Obstetrics and Gynecology.

58. Ibid.

59. National Council on Alcoholism and Drug Dependence.

60. Ewing, J.A., "Detecting Alcoholism: The CAGE Questionnaire." *Journal of the American Medical Association*, 1984.

Notes

61. "Understanding Alcohol," NIH Curriculum Supplement Series. National Institutes for Health, 2003.

62. *Global Status Report: Alcohol Policy*. World Health Organization, 2004.

63. DUI, DWI and Other State Laws. U.S. Department of Labor.

64. Ibid.

65. 2005 National Survey on Drug Use and Health: National Findings. Department of Health and Human Services. Substance Abuse and Mental Health Services Administration, Office of Applied Studies.

66. Pennebaker, James, "Writing About Emotional Experiences as a Therapeutic Process," *Psychological Science*, 1997.

67. Babyak, Blumenthal, James, et al., "Exercise Treatment for Major Depression: Maintenance of Therapeutic Benefit at 10 Months." *Psychosomatic Medicine*, 2000.

68. Rose, Amanda. "Prospective Associations of Co-Rumination With Friendship and Emotional Adjustment: Considering the Socioemotional Trade-Offs of Co-rumination," Developmental Psychology, July 2007.

69. Brody, Jane E., "The Growing Wave of Teenage Self-Injury." *The New York Times*, May 6, 2008.

INDEX

Index